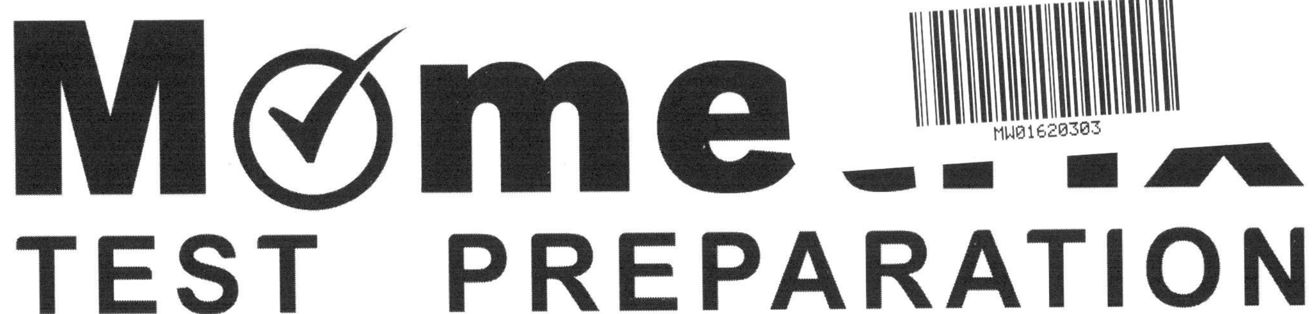

National Opticianry Competency Exam Secrets Study Guide

DEAR FUTURE EXAM SUCCESS STORY

First of all, **THANK YOU** for purchasing Mometrix study materials!

Second, congratulations! You are one of the few determined test-takers who are committed to doing whatever it takes to excel on your exam. **You have come to the right place.** We developed these study materials with one goal in mind: to deliver you the information you need in a format that's concise and easy to use.

In addition to optimizing your guide for the content of the test, we've outlined our recommended steps for breaking down the preparation process into small, attainable goals so you can make sure you stay on track.

We've also analyzed the entire test-taking process, identifying the most common pitfalls and showing how you can overcome them and be ready for any curveball the test throws you.

Standardized testing is one of the biggest obstacles on your road to success, which only increases the importance of doing well in the high-pressure, high-stakes environment of test day. Your results on this test could have a significant impact on your future, and this guide provides the information and practical advice to help you achieve your full potential on test day.

Your success is our success

We would love to hear from you! If you would like to share the story of your exam success or if you have any questions or comments in regard to our products, please contact us at **800-673-8175** or **support@mometrix.com**.

Thanks again for your business and we wish you continued success!

Sincerely,
The Mometrix Test Preparation Team

Need more help? Check out our flashcards at:
http://mometrixflashcards.com/NOCE

Written and edited by the Mometrix Exam Secrets Test Prep Team
Printed in the United States of America

TABLE OF CONTENTS

Introduction

Thank you for purchasing this resource! You have made the choice to prepare yourself for a test that could have a huge impact on your future, and this guide is designed to help you be fully ready for test day. Obviously, it's important to have a solid understanding of the test material, but you also need to be prepared for the unique environment and stressors of the test, so that you can perform to the best of your abilities.

For this purpose, the first section that appears in this guide is the **Secret Keys**. We've devoted countless hours to meticulously researching what works and what doesn't, and we've boiled down our findings to the five most impactful steps you can take to improve your performance on the test. We start at the beginning with study planning and move through the preparation process, all the way to the testing strategies that will help you get the most out of what you know when you're finally sitting in front of the test.

We recommend that you start preparing for your test as far in advance as possible. However, if you've bought this guide as a last-minute study resource and only have a few days before your test, we recommend that you skip over the first two Secret Keys since they address a long-term study plan.

If you struggle with **test anxiety**, we strongly encourage you to check out our recommendations for how you can overcome it. Test anxiety is a formidable foe, but it can be beaten, and we want to make sure you have the tools you need to defeat it.

Secret Key 1: Plan Big, Study Small

There's a lot riding on your performance. If you want to ace this test, you're going to need to keep your skills sharp and the material fresh in your mind. You need a plan that lets you review everything you need to know while still fitting in your schedule. We'll break this strategy down into three categories.

Information Organization

Start with the information you already have: the official test outline. From this, you can make a complete list of all the concepts you need to cover before the test. Organize these concepts into groups that can be studied together, and create a list of any related vocabulary you need to learn so you can brush up on any difficult terms. You'll want to keep this vocabulary list handy once you actually start studying since you may need to add to it along the way.

Time Management

Once you have your set of study concepts, decide how to spread them out over the time you have left before the test. Break your study plan into small, clear goals so you have a manageable task for each day and know exactly what you're doing. Then just focus on one small step at a time. When you manage your time this way, you don't need to spend hours at a time studying. Studying a small block of content for a short period each day helps you retain information better and avoid stressing over how much you have left to do. You can relax knowing that you have a plan to cover everything in time. In order for this strategy to be effective though, you have to start studying early and stick to your schedule. Avoid the exhaustion and futility that comes from last-minute cramming!

Study Environment

The environment you study in has a big impact on your learning. Studying in a coffee shop, while probably more enjoyable, is not likely to be as fruitful as studying in a quiet room. It's important to keep distractions to a minimum. You're only planning to study for a short block of time, so make the most of it. Don't pause to check your phone or get up to find a snack. It's also important to **avoid multitasking**. Research has consistently shown that multitasking will make your studying dramatically less effective. Your study area should also be comfortable and well-lit so you don't have the distraction of straining your eyes or sitting on an uncomfortable chair.

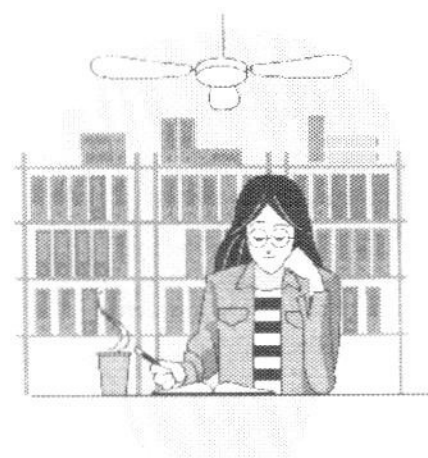

The time of day you study is also important. You want to be rested and alert. Don't wait until just before bedtime. Study when you'll be most likely to comprehend and remember. Even better, if you know what time of day your test will be, set that time aside for study. That way your brain will be used to working on that subject at that specific time and you'll have a better chance of recalling information.

Finally, it can be helpful to team up with others who are studying for the same test. Your actual studying should be done in as isolated an environment as possible, but the work of organizing the information and setting up the study plan can be divided up. In between study sessions, you can discuss with your teammates the concepts that you're all studying and quiz each other on the details. Just be sure that your teammates are as serious about the test as you are. If you find that your study time is being replaced with social time, you might need to find a new team.

Secret Key 2: Make Your Studying Count

You're devoting a lot of time and effort to preparing for this test, so you want to be absolutely certain it will pay off. This means doing more than just reading the content and hoping you can remember it on test day. It's important to make every minute of study count. There are two main areas you can focus on to make your studying count.

Retention

It doesn't matter how much time you study if you can't remember the material. You need to make sure you are retaining the concepts. To check your retention of the information you're learning, try recalling it at later times with minimal prompting. Try carrying around flashcards and glance at one or two from time to time or ask a friend who's also studying for the test to quiz you.

To enhance your retention, look for ways to put the information into practice so that you can apply it rather than simply recalling it. If you're using the information in practical ways, it will be much easier to remember. Similarly, it helps to solidify a concept in your mind if you're not only reading it to yourself but also explaining it to someone else. Ask a friend to let you teach them about a concept you're a little shaky on (or speak aloud to an imaginary audience if necessary). As you try to summarize, define, give examples, and answer your friend's questions, you'll understand the concepts better and they will stay with you longer. Finally, step back for a big picture view and ask yourself how each piece of information fits with the whole subject. When you link the different concepts together and see them working together as a whole, it's easier to remember the individual components.

Finally, practice showing your work on any multi-step problems, even if you're just studying. Writing out each step you take to solve a problem will help solidify the process in your mind, and you'll be more likely to remember it during the test.

Modality

Modality simply refers to the means or method by which you study. Choosing a study modality that fits your own individual learning style is crucial. No two people learn best in exactly the same way, so it's important to know your strengths and use them to your advantage.

For example, if you learn best by visualization, focus on visualizing a concept in your mind and draw an image or a diagram. Try color-coding your notes, illustrating them, or creating symbols that will trigger your mind to recall a learned concept. If you learn best by hearing or discussing information, find a study partner who learns the same way or read aloud to yourself. Think about how to put the information in your own words. Imagine that you are giving a lecture on the topic and record yourself so you can listen to it later.

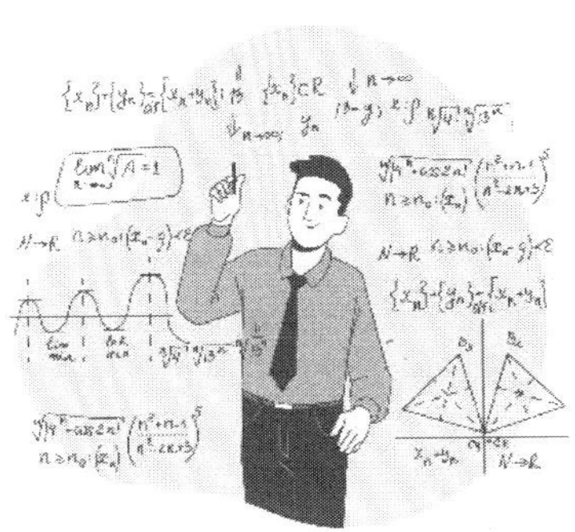

For any learning style, flashcards can be helpful. Organize the information so you can take advantage of spare moments to review. Underline key words or phrases. Use different colors for different categories. Mnemonic devices (such as creating a short list in which every item starts with the same letter) can also help with retention. Find what works best for you and use it to store the information in your mind most effectively and easily.

Secret Key 3: Practice the Right Way

Your success on test day depends not only on how many hours you put into preparing, but also on whether you prepared the right way. It's good to check along the way to see if your studying is paying off. One of the most effective ways to do this is by taking practice tests to evaluate your progress. Practice tests are useful because they show exactly where you need to improve. Every time you take a practice test, pay special attention to these three groups of questions:

- The questions you got wrong
- The questions you had to guess on, even if you guessed right
- The questions you found difficult or slow to work through

This will show you exactly what your weak areas are, and where you need to devote more study time. Ask yourself why each of these questions gave you trouble. Was it because you didn't understand the material? Was it because you didn't remember the vocabulary? Do you need more repetitions on this type of question to build speed and confidence? Dig into those questions and figure out how you can strengthen your weak areas as you go back to review the material.

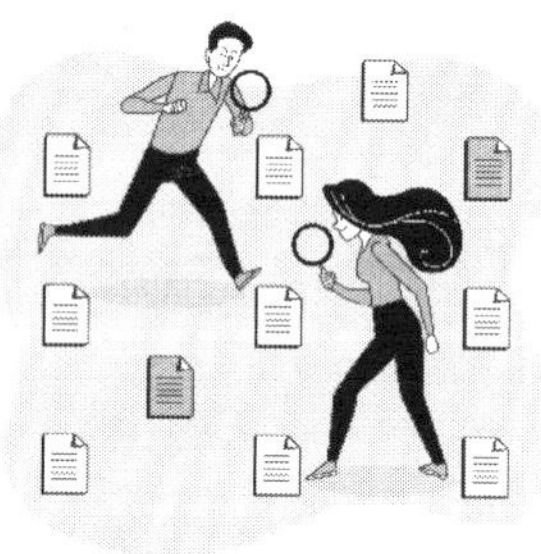

Additionally, many practice tests have a section explaining the answer choices. It can be tempting to read the explanation and think that you now have a good understanding of the concept. However, an explanation likely only covers part of the question's broader context. Even if the explanation makes perfect sense, **go back and investigate** every concept related to the question until you're positive you have a thorough understanding.

As you go along, keep in mind that the practice test is just that: practice. Memorizing these questions and answers will not be very helpful on the actual test because it is unlikely to have any of the same exact questions. If you only know the right answers to the sample questions, you won't be prepared for the real thing. **Study the concepts** until you understand them fully, and then you'll be able to answer any question that shows up on the test.

It's important to wait on the practice tests until you're ready. If you take a test on your first day of study, you may be overwhelmed by the amount of material covered and how much you need to learn. Work up to it gradually.

On test day, you'll need to be prepared for answering questions, managing your time, and using the test-taking strategies you've learned. It's a lot to balance, like a mental marathon that will have a big impact on your future. Like training for a marathon, you'll need to start slowly and work your way up. When test day arrives, you'll be ready.

Start with the strategies you've read in the first two Secret Keys—plan your course and study in the way that works best for you. If you have time, consider using multiple study resources to get different approaches to the same concepts. It can be helpful to see difficult concepts from more than one angle. Then find a good source for practice tests. Many times, the test website will suggest potential study resources or provide sample tests.

Practice Test Strategy

If you're able to find at least three practice tests, we recommend this strategy:

Untimed and Open-Book Practice

Take the first test with no time constraints and with your notes and study guide handy. Take your time and focus on applying the strategies you've learned.

Timed and Open-Book Practice

Take the second practice test open-book as well, but set a timer and practice pacing yourself to finish in time.

Timed and Closed-Book Practice

Take any other practice tests as if it were test day. Set a timer and put away your study materials. Sit at a table or desk in a quiet room, imagine yourself at the testing center, and answer questions as quickly and accurately as possible.

Keep repeating timed and closed-book tests on a regular basis until you run out of practice tests or it's time for the actual test. Your mind will be ready for the schedule and stress of test day, and you'll be able to focus on recalling the material you've learned.

Secret Key 4: Pace Yourself

Once you're fully prepared for the material on the test, your biggest challenge on test day will be managing your time. Just knowing that the clock is ticking can make you panic even if you have plenty of time left. Work on pacing yourself so you can build confidence against the time constraints of the exam. Pacing is a difficult skill to master, especially in a high-pressure environment, so **practice is vital**.

Set time expectations for your pace based on how much time is available. For example, if a section has 60 questions and the time limit is 30 minutes, you know you have to average 30 seconds or less per question in order to answer them all. Although 30 seconds is the hard limit, set 25 seconds per question as your goal, so you reserve extra time to spend on harder questions. When you budget extra time for the harder questions, you no longer have any reason to stress when those questions take longer to answer.

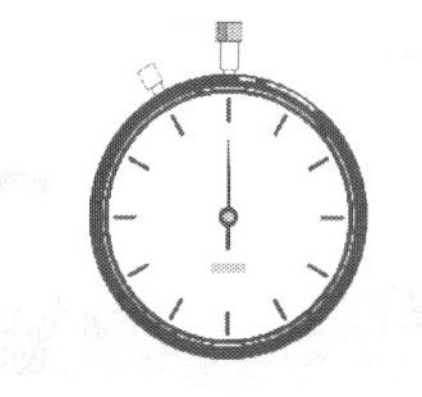

Don't let this time expectation distract you from working through the test at a calm, steady pace, but keep it in mind so you don't spend too much time on any one question. Recognize that taking extra time on one question you don't understand may keep you from answering two that you do understand later in the test. If your time limit for a question is up and you're still not sure of the answer, mark it and move on, and come back to it later if the time and the test format allow. If the testing format doesn't allow you to return to earlier questions, just make an educated guess; then put it out of your mind and move on.

On the easier questions, be careful not to rush. It may seem wise to hurry through them so you have more time for the challenging ones, but it's not worth missing one if you know the concept and just didn't take the time to read the question fully. Work efficiently but make sure you understand the question and have looked at all of the answer choices, since more than one may seem right at first.

Even if you're paying attention to the time, you may find yourself a little behind at some point. You should speed up to get back on track, but do so wisely. Don't panic; just take a few seconds less on each question until you're caught up. Don't guess without thinking, but do look through the answer choices and eliminate any you know are wrong. If you can get down to two choices, it is often worthwhile to guess from those. Once you've chosen an answer, move on and don't dwell on any that you skipped or had to hurry through. If a question was taking too long, chances are it was one of the harder ones, so you weren't as likely to get it right anyway.

On the other hand, if you find yourself getting ahead of schedule, it may be beneficial to slow down a little. The more quickly you work, the more likely you are to make a careless mistake that will affect your score. You've budgeted time for each question, so don't be afraid to spend that time. Practice an efficient but careful pace to get the most out of the time you have.

Secret Key 5: Have a Plan for Guessing

When you're taking the test, you may find yourself stuck on a question. Some of the answer choices seem better than others, but you don't see the one answer choice that is obviously correct. What do you do?

The scenario described above is very common, yet most test takers have not effectively prepared for it. Developing and practicing a plan for guessing may be one of the single most effective uses of your time as you get ready for the exam.

In developing your plan for guessing, there are three questions to address:

- When should you start the guessing process?
- How should you narrow down the choices?
- Which answer should you choose?

When to Start the Guessing Process

Unless your plan for guessing is to select C every time (which, despite its merits, is not what we recommend), you need to leave yourself enough time to apply your answer elimination strategies. Since you have a limited amount of time for each question, that means that if you're going to give yourself the best shot at guessing correctly, you have to decide quickly whether or not you will guess.

Of course, the best-case scenario is that you don't have to guess at all, so first, see if you can answer the question based on your knowledge of the subject and basic reasoning skills. Focus on the key words in the question and try to jog your memory of related topics. Give yourself a chance to bring the knowledge to mind, but once you realize that you don't have (or you can't access) the knowledge you need to answer the question, it's time to start the guessing process.

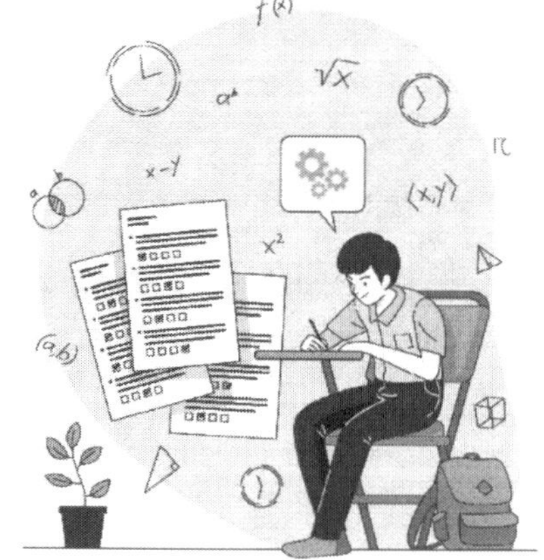

It's almost always better to start the guessing process too early than too late. It only takes a few seconds to remember something and answer the question from knowledge. Carefully eliminating wrong answer choices takes longer. Plus, going through the process of eliminating answer choices can actually help jog your memory.

Summary: Start the guessing process as soon as you decide that you can't answer the question based on your knowledge.

How to Narrow Down the Choices

The next chapter in this book (**Test-Taking Strategies**) includes a wide range of strategies for how to approach questions and how to look for answer choices to eliminate. You will definitely want to read those carefully, practice them, and figure out which ones work best for you. Here though, we're going to address a mindset rather than a particular strategy.

Your odds of guessing an answer correctly depend on how many options you are choosing from.

Number of options left	5	4	3	2	1
Odds of guessing correctly	20%	25%	33%	50%	100%

You can see from this chart just how valuable it is to be able to eliminate incorrect answers and make an educated guess, but there are two things that many test takers do that cause them to miss out on the benefits of guessing:

- Accidentally eliminating the correct answer
- Selecting an answer based on an impression

We'll look at the first one here, and the second one in the next section.

To avoid accidentally eliminating the correct answer, we recommend a thought exercise called **the $5 challenge**. In this challenge, you only eliminate an answer choice from contention if you are willing to bet $5 on it being wrong. Why $5? Five dollars is a small but not insignificant amount of money. It's an amount you could afford to lose but wouldn't want to throw away. And while losing $5 once might not hurt too much, doing it twenty times will set you back $100. In the same way, each small decision you make—eliminating a choice here, guessing on a question there—won't by itself impact your score very much, but when you put them all together, they can make a big difference. By holding each answer choice elimination decision to a higher standard, you can reduce the risk of accidentally eliminating the correct answer.

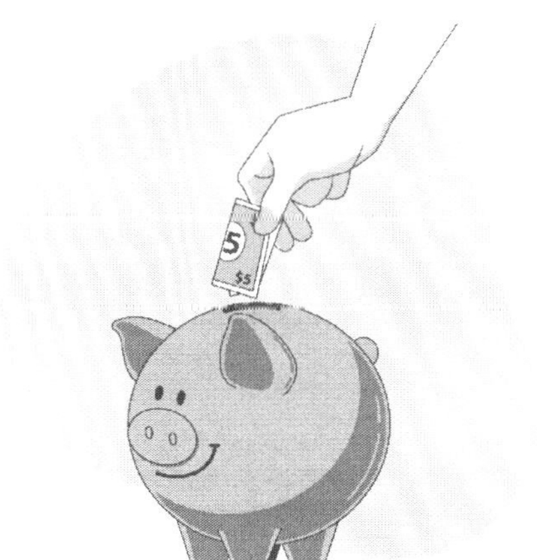

The $5 challenge can also be applied in a positive sense: If you are willing to bet $5 that an answer choice *is* correct, go ahead and mark it as correct.

Summary: Only eliminate an answer choice if you are willing to bet $5 that it is wrong.

Which Answer to Choose

You're taking the test. You've run into a hard question and decided you'll have to guess. You've eliminated all the answer choices you're willing to bet $5 on. Now you have to pick an answer. Why do we even need to talk about this? Why can't you just pick whichever one you feel like when the time comes?

The answer to these questions is that if you don't come into the test with a plan, you'll rely on your impression to select an answer choice, and if you do that, you risk falling into a trap. The test writers know that everyone who takes their test will be guessing on some of the questions, so they intentionally write wrong answer choices to seem plausible. You still have to pick an answer though, and if the wrong answer choices are designed to look right, how can you ever be sure that you're not falling for their trap? The best solution we've found to this dilemma is to take the decision out of your hands entirely. Here is the process we recommend:

Once you've eliminated any choices that you are confident (willing to bet $5) are wrong, select the first remaining choice as your answer.

Whether you choose to select the first remaining choice, the second, or the last, the important thing is that you use some preselected standard. Using this approach guarantees that you will not be enticed into selecting an answer choice that looks right, because you are not basing your decision on how the answer choices look.

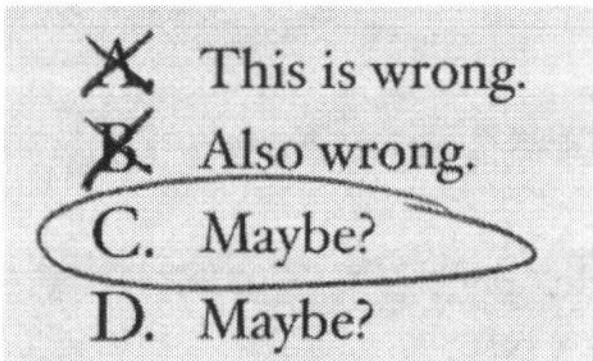

This is not meant to make you question your knowledge. Instead, it is to help you recognize the difference between your knowledge and your impressions. There's a huge difference between thinking an answer is right because of what you know, and thinking an answer is right because it looks or sounds like it should be right.

Summary: To ensure that your selection is appropriately random, make a predetermined selection from among all answer choices you have not eliminated.

Test-Taking Strategies

This section contains a list of test-taking strategies that you may find helpful as you work through the test. By taking what you know and applying logical thought, you can maximize your chances of answering any question correctly!

It is very important to realize that every question is different and every person is different: no single strategy will work on every question, and no single strategy will work for every person. That's why we've included all of them here, so you can try them out and determine which ones work best for different types of questions and which ones work best for you.

Question Strategies

✓ Read Carefully

Read the question and the answer choices carefully. Don't miss the question because you misread the terms. You have plenty of time to read each question thoroughly and make sure you understand what is being asked. Yet a happy medium must be attained, so don't waste too much time. You must read carefully and efficiently.

✓ Contextual Clues

Look for contextual clues. If the question includes a word you are not familiar with, look at the immediate context for some indication of what the word might mean. Contextual clues can often give you all the information you need to decipher the meaning of an unfamiliar word. Even if you can't determine the meaning, you may be able to narrow down the possibilities enough to make a solid guess at the answer to the question.

✓ Prefixes

If you're having trouble with a word in the question or answer choices, try dissecting it. Take advantage of every clue that the word might include. Prefixes can be a huge help. Usually, they allow you to determine a basic meaning. *Pre-* means before, *post-* means after, *pro-* is positive, *de-* is negative. From prefixes, you can get an idea of the general meaning of the word and try to put it into context.

✓ Hedge Words

Watch out for critical hedge words, such as *likely, may, can, sometimes, often, almost, mostly, usually, generally, rarely*, and *sometimes*. Question writers insert these hedge phrases to cover every possibility. Often an answer choice will be wrong simply because it leaves no room for exception. Be on guard for answer choices that have definitive words such as *exactly* and *always*.

✓ Switchback Words

Stay alert for *switchbacks*. These are the words and phrases frequently used to alert you to shifts in thought. The most common switchback words are *but*, *although*, and *however*. Others include *nevertheless*, *on the other hand*, *even though*, *while*, *in spite of*, *despite*, and *regardless of*. Switchback words are important to catch because they can change the direction of the question or an answer choice.

✓ Face Value

When in doubt, use common sense. Accept the situation in the problem at face value. Don't read too much into it. These problems will not require you to make wild assumptions. If you have to go beyond creativity and warp time or space in order to have an answer choice fit the question, then you should move on and consider the other answer choices. These are normal problems rooted in reality. The applicable relationship or explanation may not be readily apparent, but it is there for you to figure out. Use your common sense to interpret anything that isn't clear.

Answer Choice Strategies

✓ Answer Selection

The most thorough way to pick an answer choice is to identify and eliminate wrong answers until only one is left, then confirm it is the correct answer. Sometimes an answer choice may immediately seem right, but be careful. The test writers will usually put more than one reasonable answer choice on each question, so take a second to read all of them and make sure that the other choices are not equally obvious. As long as you have time left, it is better to read every answer choice than to pick the first one that looks right without checking the others.

✓ Answer Choice Families

An answer choice family consists of two (in rare cases, three) answer choices that are very similar in construction and cannot all be true at the same time. If you see two answer choices that are direct opposites or parallels, one of them is usually the correct answer. For instance, if one answer choice says that quantity x increases and another either says that quantity x decreases (opposite) or says that quantity y increases (parallel), then those answer choices would fall into the same family. An answer choice that doesn't match the construction of the answer choice family is more likely to be incorrect. Most questions will not have answer choice families, but when they do appear, you should be prepared to recognize them.

✓ Eliminate Answers

Eliminate answer choices as soon as you realize they are wrong, but make sure you consider all possibilities. If you are eliminating answer choices and realize that the last one you are left with is also wrong, don't panic. Start over and consider each choice again. There may be something you missed the first time that you will realize on the second pass.

✅ AVOID FACT TRAPS

Don't be distracted by an answer choice that is factually true but doesn't answer the question. You are looking for the choice that answers the question. Stay focused on what the question is asking for so you don't accidentally pick an answer that is true but incorrect. Always go back to the question and make sure the answer choice you've selected actually answers the question and is not merely a true statement.

✅ EXTREME STATEMENTS

In general, you should avoid answers that put forth extreme actions as standard practice or proclaim controversial ideas as established fact. An answer choice that states the "process should be used in certain situations, if…" is much more likely to be correct than one that states the "process should be discontinued completely." The first is a calm rational statement and doesn't even make a definitive, uncompromising stance, using a hedge word *if* to provide wiggle room, whereas the second choice is far more extreme.

✅ BENCHMARK

As you read through the answer choices and you come across one that seems to answer the question well, mentally select that answer choice. This is not your final answer, but it's the one that will help you evaluate the other answer choices. The one that you selected is your benchmark or standard for judging each of the other answer choices. Every other answer choice must be compared to your benchmark. That choice is correct until proven otherwise by another answer choice beating it. If you find a better answer, then that one becomes your new benchmark. Once you've decided that no other choice answers the question as well as your benchmark, you have your final answer.

✅ PREDICT THE ANSWER

Before you even start looking at the answer choices, it is often best to try to predict the answer. When you come up with the answer on your own, it is easier to avoid distractions and traps because you will know exactly what to look for. The right answer choice is unlikely to be word-for-word what you came up with, but it should be a close match. Even if you are confident that you have the right answer, you should still take the time to read each option before moving on.

General Strategies

✅ TOUGH QUESTIONS

If you are stumped on a problem or it appears too hard or too difficult, don't waste time. Move on! Remember though, if you can quickly check for obviously incorrect answer choices, your chances of guessing correctly are greatly improved. Before you completely give up, at least try to knock out a couple of possible answers. Eliminate what you can and then guess at the remaining answer choices before moving on.

✓ Check Your Work

Since you will probably not know every term listed and the answer to every question, it is important that you get credit for the ones that you do know. Don't miss any questions through careless mistakes. If at all possible, try to take a second to look back over your answer selection and make sure you've selected the correct answer choice and haven't made a costly careless mistake (such as marking an answer choice that you didn't mean to mark). This quick double check should more than pay for itself in caught mistakes for the time it costs.

✓ Pace Yourself

It's easy to be overwhelmed when you're looking at a page full of questions; your mind is confused and full of random thoughts, and the clock is ticking down faster than you would like. Calm down and maintain the pace that you have set for yourself. Especially as you get down to the last few minutes of the test, don't let the small numbers on the clock make you panic. As long as you are on track by monitoring your pace, you are guaranteed to have time for each question.

✓ Don't Rush

It is very easy to make errors when you are in a hurry. Maintaining a fast pace in answering questions is pointless if it makes you miss questions that you would have gotten right otherwise. Test writers like to include distracting information and wrong answers that seem right. Taking a little extra time to avoid careless mistakes can make all the difference in your test score. Find a pace that allows you to be confident in the answers that you select.

✓ Keep Moving

Panicking will not help you pass the test, so do your best to stay calm and keep moving. Taking deep breaths and going through the answer elimination steps you practiced can help to break through a stress barrier and keep your pace.

Final Notes

The combination of a solid foundation of content knowledge and the confidence that comes from practicing your plan for applying that knowledge is the key to maximizing your performance on test day. As your foundation of content knowledge is built up and strengthened, you'll find that the strategies included in this chapter become more and more effective in helping you quickly sift through the distractions and traps of the test to isolate the correct answer.

Now that you're preparing to move forward into the test content chapters of this book, be sure to keep your goal in mind. As you read, think about how you will be able to apply this information on the test. If you've already seen sample questions for the test and you have an idea of the question format and style, try to come up with questions of your own that you can answer based on what you're reading. This will give you valuable practice applying your knowledge in the same ways you can expect to on test day.

Good luck and good studying!

Ophthalmic Optics

VISIBLE LIGHT

Visible light is the small portion in the middle of the **electromagnetic spectrum** that our eyes can perceive. It has longer wavelengths than radio uses, but shorter wavelengths than X-rays. The majority of the light that we see falls between wavelengths of 400 and 700 nanometers (nm), with red light on the longer end and violet light on the shorter end. Light waves longer than what we see as red are called **infrared**, whereas light waves shorter than our visible range are referred to as **ultraviolet**.

WAVELENGTH LEAST HARMFUL THE EYE

Light on the red end of the spectrum has the longest wavelength and is the least likely to cause harm to the eye. Light on the opposite end of the visible spectrum, the shorter wavelengths, is much more likely to cause harm to the eye's internal and external structures. Prolonged exposure to **high-energy violet** light can, over time, degrade the light-receptor cells in the retina, whereas ultraviolet light (much of it not visible to the human eye) can cause immediate damage to the eye's cornea and lens. Witness the steady yellowing of an automobile headlamp lens, over time, which is also caused by prolonged ultraviolet exposure.

ULTRAVIOLET LIGHT

Ultraviolet light is generally described as that range from 400 nm, at the very shortest wavelengths we can see, down to about 100 nm. The longest of those wavelengths, between 400 and 320 nm, is the least harmful and is called **UVA**. **UVB** light has wavelengths between 320 and 290 nm, and it is responsible for sunburns and many skin cancers. **UVC**, the shortest wavelength (between 290 and 100 nm), is extremely harmful to all kinds of life; it is sometimes used to destroy microorganisms in water or food or on surgical instruments. Fortunately, these wavelengths are almost all absorbed by the Earth's atmosphere. (There is also an **extreme ultraviolet** range, from 100 nm down to 10 nm, but this type of radiation can only travel through a vacuum and is completely absorbed by our atmosphere.)

REFRACTION OF LIGHT

When a ray of light passes from one medium (such as air) into a denser medium (such as a glass lens), striking at any angle other than 90 degrees, it is bent to one side, which is the essence of what we call **refraction**. The degree to which it is bent depends on the **angle of incidence**, meaning the angle at which the light encounters the barrier between the two materials. A steeper angle of incidence will result in a steeper angle of refraction. This concept can easily be illustrated by standing a straw in a clear glass of water and observing how the light reflected off the water-covered portion of the straw will make it appear to be displaced, relative to the end of the straw that is above the water.

Effect of a Denser Medium on the Speed of Light

The speed of light in a vacuum is roughly 186,282 miles per second (mps). Our atmosphere diminishes this speed only slightly, to about 186,220 mps. But water, a much denser material, slows the speed of light down to about 140,000 mps. This drop in speed is what causes the light to be bent, and any image seen through the water will be displaced. The more the higher density medium slows down the speed of the light passing through it, the greater the light will be bent. (A typical crown-glass lens will slow the speed of light down to about 122,500 mps.)

Effect on Light Passing Through a Plus or a Minus Lens

When light passes through a lens that is thicker in the center (commonly called a plus lens), the light rays toward the edges of the lens are bent inward, causing them to **converge** to a common point at a specific distance from the lens. With a lens shaped the other way around, thinner in the center than at the edges (commonly called a minus lens), the light rays toward the edges of the lens are bent outward, causing them to **diverge** rather than converge. Thus, whereas a plus lens will produce a projected image of the light source, a minus lens will only scatter the light, producing a dim, diffuse shadow.

Diopter

The basic unit of measurement of refractive power is called the **diopter**. It is defined as the amount of refractive power required to displace a ray of light by 1 cm at a distance of 1 m from the lens. This is most easily measured using a simple prism lens and passing the coherent beam of a laser through it. A one-diopter prism will bend the laser beam just enough that at a distance of 1 m from the prism, the point of light will deviate by 1 cm.

Focal Length of a Lens

When light passes through a lens and converges to a point, the distance from the lens to the focused image is referred to as the **focal length** of the lens. Stronger lenses have shorter focal lengths than weaker lenses, meaning the image will come to a focus further from a weaker lens than it would with a stronger lens. This is easily measurable with a plus lens, which causes the light rays to converge, but minus lenses also have a **focal point**, known as a virtual focal point, located at a corresponding distance behind the lens, rather than in front of it. This can be conceptualized by thinking of following the divergence in reverse, to a theoretical point behind the lens from which the divergence emanates. Needless to say, it is much easier to measure the focal length of a plus lens.

Relationship Between Lens Power and Focal Length

The dioptric power of any lens has an inverse relationship to its focal length. Whereas a one-diopter lens will have a focal length of 1 m, a two-diopter lens will have a focal length of 0.5 m, a four-diopter lens will have a focal length of only 0.25 m, and so on. Thus, the two can be considered reciprocals of each other. Mathematically, the formula is $D = 1/F$, or conversely, $F = 1/D$, where D is the power in diopters and F is the focal length in meters.

Vertex Distance and Final Visual Correction of Patient's Eyewear

When an optometrist determines an eyeglass prescription, he measures it with the phoropter lenses at about 12–15 mm from the surface of the eye. This is known as the **vertex distance**. If the completed eyewear deviates from that distance enough and the lenses are sufficiently powerful, a stronger or weaker lens may be required in order to give the patient an **effective power** equal to the written prescription.

In general, a minus lens that is moved closer to the eye will produce a greater effective power for the patient, whereas moving it away will weaken the effective power. The phenomenon works in the exact reverse for a plus lens.

The formula for determining how much the lens power must be compensated for this effect is $Dc = D / (1 - dD)$, where D is the written power, d is the vertex deviation in meters, and Dc is the resulting change in effective power, in raw terms. For a minus lens moved closer, the formula will render the actual effective power at that range and you would subtract the deviation to get the necessary compensated power. When moving it further away, the formula renders the compensated power. The opposite is true for plus powers.

Prescription Elements

The three main elements of every prescription are **sphere power**, **cylinder power**, and **axis**.

Sphere power is a measure of how **myopic** (nearsighted) or **hyperopic** (farsighted) a patient's vision is, with plus lenses correcting hyperopia and minus lenses correcting myopia. Plano, or zero, indicates that the patient is neither myopic nor hyperopic, but **emmetropic**.

Cylinder power is a measure of how much **astigmatism** is affecting the vision. Astigmatism is a defect of the cornea that causes the light to be bent in more than one direction.

Axis is the orientation of the cylinder power, along a line at the given angle between 0 and 180.

The designations OD and OS stand for **oculus dexter** and **oculus sinister**, meaning right eye and left eye. (Dexter is Latin for right, or favorable, whereas sinister meant unfavorable or injurious. Left-handed people were once thought to be possessed by evil spirits.) OU is seen when the two eyes share the same value, and it stands for **oculus uterque**.

Forms of Prescriptions

Prescriptions are written either in **minus-cylinder** format or **plus-cylinder** format. The former, where the cylinder power will always be a negative value, is the more commonly used format, employed by lens manufacturers, preferred by optical labs, and used by most optometrists. The latter format is typically used by ophthalmologists. In that form, the cylinder power will be a positive value. Its use by ophthalmologists dates back to early eye surgeries, where an incision in the cornea would leave a scar across the cornea, which became the astigmatic axis. Today, the format no longer serves this logical purpose, and its continued use is simply a symbolic way of differentiating the M.D. from the O.D. Manufacturing of lenses with actual plus cylinder has been abandoned, partially due to its increased cost, and all modern lenses are made in minus cylinder.

Simple Spherical Rx, Simple Astigmatic Rx, and Rx with Compound Spherocylindrical Correction

A spherical Rx consists of sphere power only, and it will correct simple myopia or hyperopia, shortening or extending the focal length of the eye so that light comes to a focus on the retina.

An astigmatic Rx, in which the sphere power is plano but there are values for cylinder and axis, will correct for **asphericity** of the cornea, which causes the light to focus on the retina as a smeared blob rather than a point. The lens will have two back curvatures at 90 degrees from each other, precisely counteracting the aspheric corneal defect and causing all of the light through an astigmatic cornea to be redirected to a point focus.

A spherocylinder Rx, with all three elements containing values other than zero, corrects for both refractive errors at the same time, correcting the focal length of the lens and cornea as well as the cornea's asphericity to bring the light to a crisp point of focus on the retina.

Archaic Format for Written Prescriptions

These days, most refractions are carried out using a **phoropter**, where the patient sits in a chair with this complex instrument against his face. The doctor proceeds to use patient input to refine the Rx further and further. The resulting prescription will be written in the three- or four-element form we are all familiar with.

At one time, refractions were routinely carried out using a set of trial lenses in a trial frame. During this era, the **Jackson crossed-cylinder** method was the accepted way of establishing a patient's astigmatism. It involved using two cylindrical trial lenses at 90 degrees from each other to pinpoint the prescription. The resulting Rx, known simply as the crossed-cylinder format, would look something like this: −2.00 X 160 ^ −3.25 X 070, and it would be translated into modern format as - 2.00 - 1.25 X 070 (or −3.25 +1.25 X 160).

Function of an Add Power

The eye is formed with the ability to create on-demand changes in focus from distant objects to those as close as a foot or less at birth. As the eye ages, it gradually loses this ability, creating less and less magnification for near objects. This condition is called **presbyopia**. When this advances enough to prevent clear vision at a normal reading distance (usually 16 inches), the optometrist will begin including an **add power** as the final element of the Rx. This extra power (generally located only near the bottom of a multifocal lens) will produce sufficient additional magnification to restore comfortable near viewing, making up for the age-related deficit.

Common Written Format of Prescribed Prism

Prescribed prism is always given in diopters and direction, for each lens on which it is desired. For example, the OD (right eye) prescription will read as +1.25 −0.50 X 115 3.0 BD, which indicates that there should be three diopters of prism **base down**, read in the lensometer as downward from normal center. **Base up** (BU) prism will read above center, **base in** (BI) prism will read off center toward the nose, and **base out** (BO) prism will read toward the eye's temporal edge. Prism may also be prescribed in two directions at once in the same lens, such as 3.0 BI or 2.0 BU.

Base Curve of a Lens

The term **base curve**, at its simplest, means the curve from which all other curves are calculated. In optical lens design, this commonly refers to the front curvature of the lens. The power of the lens will be determined by how the curvature(s) on the back of the lens relates to the base curve. If the curvature on the back of the lens is steeper than the base curve, the lens will have a minus power. If the curvature on the back of the lens is flatter than the base curve, then the lens will have a plus power. Equal curvatures would result in the lens power being plano, or zero.

Selecting a Base Curvature

The primary consideration when selecting a base curve is in reducing visual distortions for the patient. Any lens of the proper power, when viewing an object directly in front of it, will produce an accurate image on the patient's retina. However, that same lens, when viewing an object toward the edge of the visual field, can introduce distortions known as **off-axis astigmatism**. This results from those oblique rays being bent too much or too little when striking the edge of a lens with too much or too little curvature.

The standard rule of thumb has long been to minimize this effect by maintaining a rear lens curvature as close to −6.00 diopters as possible, closely mimicking the shape of the average cornea. Thus, a plus-power lens might be made using a steeper base curve in order to keep the rear curvature from becoming too flat, whereas a minus-power lens would use a flatter base curve to keep the rear curvature from becoming too steep. Professional opinions vary on this standard, however, especially with the advent of aspheric and free-form lenses; in many of these cases, **median** curvatures are used in calculating what is ideal, making the computation more complex.

Example 1

State which base curve you would select, and why, given the following Rx: +3.50 −1.50 X 112.

We would first find the spherical equivalent of the prescription, which is +2.75. Because the goal is an average rear curvature on the lens of

−6.00, we would begin with a nominal front curve of +6.00, which would produce a plano power lens. Add the spherical equivalent of +2.75 to the nominal +6.00, obtaining a front curvature of +8.75. This would be rounded down to the nearest available value, which is +8.25, and that would be the base curve chosen for the prescription.

Example 2

State which base curve you would select, and why, given the following Rx: −5.00 +1.00 X 016.

In this case, the first step would be to convert the prescription to minus-cylinder format, which would give us −4.00 −1.00 X 106. Then, we would find the spherical equivalent of the prescription, which is −4.50. Because the goal is an average rear curvature on the lens of −6.00, we would begin with a nominal front curve of +6.00, which would produce a plano power lens. Subtract the spherical equivalent of −4.50 from the nominal +6.00, obtaining a front curvature of +1.50. This would be rounded up to the nearest available value, which is +2.00, and that would be the base curve chosen for the prescription.

Curvatures Found on Either Surface of a Lens

The first lens curvatures were all spherical, meaning they were shaped like a slice from a perfectly round ball, or sphere. In the early 1800s, we learned that not all eyesight can be corrected with these lenses, and the concept of using cylindrical curvatures to correct astigmatism was born. By the middle of that century, opticians were learning to combine spheres and cylinders, so that one side of the lens (typically today, the rear surface) has two distinct curvatures. This is called a **toric** surface.

As cataract surgery came into being, those early patients were left requiring extremely powerful plus lenses. The search for thinner and lighter lens designs for these folks led to the concept of varying the front curvature of the lens, flattening it at the edges and making it possible to thin the lenses dramatically. These were the first **aspheric** lens designs.

With the advent of digital processing, lens curvatures can be made to vary in complex ways, on the front and back surfaces, in the interest of optimizing the patient's vision over the entire lens. When this variable curvature is introduced on an astigmatic Rx, the result is referred to as an **atoric** lens surface.

Less-Common Lens Designs for Extreme Prescriptions

Before the technology really existed to create a true aspheric lens curvature, the **lenticular** lens design was widely accepted for use with high-plus prescriptions. This featured a flat carrier edge with a small central portion of +12.00 to +16.00 diopters. Often, the plano-based edge would end up as part of the finished lens, making for an odd appearance. But it did accomplish the goal of being lighter in weight than a full-field +12.00 lens would have been.

Prior to the development of the thinner lens materials we have today, the only solution for very high minus lenses was to make them biconcave, sometimes known as **myodiscs**. In these lenses, the extreme high minus power was achieved by simply factoring in the negative base curve. A lens with a −10.00 front curvature could have a −12.00 curvature ground into the back, for a surface power of −22.00 D.

Aspheric Base Curvature

An aspheric base curvature produces a lens with full prescribed power in the central visual field but weakening toward the edges. Early versions of these designs (such as the Welsh Four-Drop) were first used on the high-plus lenses of **aphakic** patients, following early cataract surgeries, in order to reduce the lenses' thickness and weight. This is still the most common benefit sought in using aspherics, although it is now rare to encounter a fully aphakic patient. Any plus lens can be made thinner and lighter by using an aspheric front curve, even if the Rx is only a +2.00.

Magnification, always a problem for hyperopic patients, can also be addressed with an aspheric lens. By flattening the lens shape significantly, the front surface is moved closer to the eye, eliminating much of the **image swim** experienced by the patient, as well as the poor cosmetics of greatly magnified eyes.

With high-power minus lenses, aspheric designs can be employed in the opposite direction, steepening an overly flat lens at the edges. This has an obvious benefit in reducing edge thickness, but it also can reduce the off-axis astigmatism of such lenses, producing clearer vision away from the center of the visual field.

Evolution of Overall Lens Design

Optical lens grinding began around the 13th century, with early opticians using trial and error to create eyeglass lenses that benefited their patients. By Galileo's day (around 1600), fine-enough optics were being produced to allow the invention of the microscope and the telescope. But these lenses were generally biconvex or biconcave spheres (either protruding outward or hollowed inward on both surfaces), or else they were plano on one side.

In order to better accommodate the shape of the eye, as well as improving the visual optics, the convex-concave lens came into use. This lens has the familiar shape we all know, curved outward in front and inward in back. Due to its likeness to the way water in a glass will curve upward at the edges, it was named the **meniscus** lens design.

Corrected-Curve Lens

One of the goals of modern lens design is to minimize off-axis distortion by keeping the back surface of the lens close to the curvature of the cornea. In practice, this can be a difficult juggling act, because traditional lens grinding procedures are constrained by a limited selection of base curvatures to choose from. This means that as the Rx increases, there will be a stepping-off point where a different base curve must be chosen; thus, the back curvature could not always be ideal because it was enslaved to the choice of base curves. With the advent of more modern lens-casting techniques, finished lenses became available in an almost unlimited array of front curvatures, making it possible to vary the base curve at will in order to keep the rear curvature more or less constant. This was called **corrected-curve** lens design. The original concept has been taken to a much higher level now that we have digital lens processing that can produce even multifocal lenses of any conceivable curvature.

Relationship of Lens Material to its Refractive Capability

The relative ability of a material to bend light as it passes through is called its **refractive index**. The standard used most commonly in quick calculations is a refractive index of 1.5, meaning that light in a vacuum travels 1.5 times the speed of light through the lens material. (In actuality, the refractive index of a plastic lens is roughly 1.49 whereas that of glass is about 1.52.) As the refractive index goes up, the light passing through is slowed down further and bent more sharply. What this means in practical terms is that a thinner lens with a higher index of refraction will focus light equally as well as a thicker one with a lower index. Thus, materials with higher indices of refraction can be used to reduce the thickness and weight of stronger prescriptions.

Effects of Lens Material on Optical Clarity

With all the choices of lens materials available today, it is important to understand their relationship to optical clarity. Thinner lens materials may improve the cosmetic appearance of the eyeglasses, but usually at the cost of rainbow-causing dispersion and higher reflectivity. There is a scale of optical clarity that was developed by German physicist Ernst Abbe, in the late 1800s, which is still in use today; it is referred to as the **Abbe value** of a lens material. Higher values are best, with ordinary glass and plastic near the top of the list at 53 and 49 respectively. Once the value drops below 45 (the Abbe value of the average cornea), the quality of the resulting image begins to suffer, with rainbows forming at the edges of the visual field and less light overall passing through the lens (up to 15% is reflected away, by the thinnest lens materials). For all of its other advantages, **polycarbonate** has one of the worst Abbe values, at about 31, making it a poor choice for any patient seeking optimum clarity.

Deducing Power of a Lens by Measuring Its Curvatures

The relationship of the front curvature of a lens to its back curvature is what gives the lens its power. Algebraically combining the two measured curves (which can be determined using a simple lens clock) will render the power of the lens.

The math for this calculation gets very complicated only when the refractive index of a given material is factored in, because the same curvatures will produce very different powers with different indices. But assuming a refractive index of 1.5 (close to that of glass or plastic), the calculation remains a simple exercise in addition and subtraction. A lens with a base curve of +6.25 and a rear surface curvature measured at −6.75 will produce power of −0.50 diopters. A lens with a base curve of +7.25 and measured rear curves of −5.00 and −6.50 will be a +2.25 lens with a −1.50 cylinder.

Calculating the Surface Power of a Lens

Example 1

Calculate the surface power of a lens that measures +4.25 on the front and −6.00 and −8.00 on the back side.

We must first combine the front curve value with the lower of the two back curve values: 4.25 − 6.00 = −1.75. Next, we compare the back curve values and take the difference between the two, in absolute value: 8.00 − 6.00 = 2.00. This means that the cylinder power of the back side is −2.00, and the total surface Rx of the lens becomes −1.75 −2.00, based on a refractive index of 1.50.

Example 2

Calculate the surface power of a lens that measures +8.37 on the front and −5.87 and −9.12 on the back side.

We must first combine the front curve value with the lower of the two back curve values: +8.37 −5.87 = +2.50. Next, we compare the back curve values and take the difference between the two, in absolute value: 9.12 − 5.87 = 3.25. This means that the cylinder power of the back side is −3.25, and the total surface Rx of the lens becomes +2.50 −3.25, based on a refractive index of 1.50.

Spherical Equivalent

When a prescription contains a cylinder power, there will be two different resulting powers at right axes to each other. But sometimes it is useful to temporarily combine the two powers into what is known as a spherical equivalent. This is essentially the median power of the prescription. It is obtained by taking half of the cylinder power and adding it to the sphere power. (Some sources advise completely ignoring cylinder powers of 0.75 and below.)

The main use for calculating a spherical equivalent is in base curve selection. Using that number as a guide, one can determine which base curve is optimal for keeping the rear curves closest to the desired standard of −6.00. The calculation also comes into play during the fitting of spherical contact lenses, when the patient is unlikely to tolerate a toric lens.

Example 1

Calculate the spherical equivalent of the following Rx:

−5.50 −3.25 X 087

In order to find the spherical equivalent, we must first halve the cylinder power, which in this case produces the unwieldy number of −1.625, which we will round down to −1.62. Combine this number with the−5.50 sphere power to obtain −7.12. This is the spherical equivalent of the prescription.

Example 2

Calculate the spherical equivalent of the following Rx:

−0.50 +1.00 X 093

In this example, we must first transpose into minus-cylinder format, giving us a new prescription of +0.50 −1.00 X 003. Then, in order to find the spherical equivalent, we must halve the cylinder power, which in this case gives us −0.50. Combine this number with the +0.50 sphere power to obtain zero. The spherical equivalent of this prescription is plano.

Determining Effective Lens Power in One Specific Direction

Often, it will be important to know the power of a spherocylinder lens along one particular axis. For example, a lens with a sphere power of plano but a cylinder of −3.00 at an axis of 180 will have an effective power of zero horizontally, but −3.00 vertically, or in the 90th meridian. This means that the lens has an infinite margin for pupillary distance (PD) error, but only a 1.0 mm margin of error for vertical imbalance. In the opposite case, in which the axis is at 90 degrees, the full −3.00 power falls along the 180 meridian, meaning that the PD error could only be about 1.0 mm, but the vertical imbalance only has to be within one-third of a diopter.

To determine the power along a specific meridian, a portion of the cylinder power is combined with the sphere power, up to 100% at 90 degrees from the axis. The cylinder power's total effect will depend on the beginning sphere power. For instance, a lens of +1.00 −2.00 X 180 will have an effective power of +1.00 at 180, −1.00 in the 90th meridian, and plano in the 45th meridian.

Determining the Power in the 90th Meridian

Determine the power in the 90th meridian, given the following Rx:

−2.25 −2.50 X 135

Given that the axis is **oblique** in this case (not close to 90 or 180), the full cylinder power is not felt in either the horizontal or vertical meridian. At either of those, only partial cylinder power will come into play. Specifically, because the axis is 45 degrees away from the vertical, 50% of the cylinder power will be effective at 90. Therefore, we combine the sphere power of −2.25 with 50% of the cylinder power, or −1.25, to obtain a power in the 90th meridian of −3.50.

Transposing Either a Plus- or Minus-Cylinder Prescription into the Opposite Form

Transposition of an Rx from one format to another is done in three distinct steps. First, the sphere and cylinder powers are combined algebraically, and the result becomes the new sphere power. Next, the sign of the cylinder power is changed from minus to plus (or plus to minus). Finally, the cylinder axis is inverted 90 degrees, by moving it either +90 or −90 to create a new value between 0 and 180. Thus, the prescription +2.25 −3.50 X 47 becomes −1.25 +3.50 X 137.

Because lens manufacturers, labs, and most opticians and optometrists work in minus-cylinder, plus-cylinder prescriptions are generally converted to minus-cylinder prior to doing anything with them. This common process is known as **flat transposition**.

Example 1

Transpose the following Rx into minus-cylinder format:

−2.00 +1.75 X 083

It is common for an ophthalmologist to give the optician an Rx in plus-cylinder format. Because most stock lenses are found in minus-cylinder, or in order to reduce the likelihood of error at the lab, it is usually advisable to convert the Rx into minus-cylinder format prior to ordering lenses.

First, the sphere and cylinder powers are combined algebraically, and the result becomes the new sphere power of −0.25. Next, the sign of the cylinder power is changed from plus to minus. Finally, the cylinder axis is inverted 90 degrees, to 173. Thus, this prescription becomes −0.25 −1.75 X 173.

Example 2

Transpose the following keratoconic Rx into minus-cylinder format:

+2.00 +4.75 X 012 add +2.25

This Rx is typical of that prescribed to a patient with keratoconus, which is a common reason why a patient might see an ophthalmologist rather than an optometrist.

First, the sphere and cylinder powers are combined algebraically, and the result becomes the new sphere power of +6.75. Next, the sign of the cylinder power is changed from plus to minus. Finally, the cylinder axis is inverted 90 degrees, to 102. The add power is left alone. Thus, this prescription becomes +6.75 −4.75 X 102 add +2.25.

Example 3

Transpose the following Rx into plus-cylinder format for use by an ophthalmologist: +2.25 −2.75 X 118 add +2.50.

When reading a pair of glasses prior to an ophthalmology exam, the doctor may wish to see the prescription in the same format within which he typically works. Thus, it may become necessary in such cases to transcribe the Rx into plus-cylinder format.

First, the sphere and cylinder powers are combined algebraically, and the result becomes the new sphere power of −0.50. Next, the sign of the cylinder power is changed from minus to plus. Finally, the cylinder axis is inverted 90 degrees, to 28. The add power is left alone. Thus, this prescription becomes −0.50 +2.75 X 028 add +2.50.

Example 4

Transpose the following Rx into a near-vision-only prescription:

−1.25 −1.50 X 016 add +1.75

There are times when a patient needs a dedicated pair of reading glasses, made to his exact prescription. These can be very useful for prolonged reading, or for any hobby that requires close-up work for any length of time.

In this case, the sphere power and the add power are combined. The new resulting sphere power becomes +0.50, making the new near-vision Rx +0.50 −1.50 X 016.

Example 5

Transpose the following Rx into a near-vision-only prescription:

+0.75 +2.75 X 167 add +2.50

In this example, the prescription has come from an ophthalmologist's office, and it must first be transposed into minus-cylinder format. The sphere and cylinder powers are combined to make +3.50, the sign of the cylinder is changed from plus to minus, and the axis is inverted 90 degrees to 77, to give us a new Rx of +3.50 −2.75 X 077 add +2.50.

After that, the sphere power and the add power are combined. The new resulting sphere power becomes +6.00, making the new near-vision Rx +6.00 −2.75 X 077.

Converting a Prescription into an Intermediate-Only Prescription

Convert the following Rx into an intermediate-only prescription:

−0.50 −1.25 X 004 add +1.50

In this case, the patient is seeking a pair of glasses for prolonged work at a computer monitor or for a musical hobby such as playing the piano. A full near-vision prescription would be too strong in this case because the intended viewing range is more like 30 inches, or arm's length.

For this use, we will use half of the prescribed add power and combine it with the sphere power, to give us +0.25. Thus, the new intermediate-only Rx becomes +0.25 −1.25 X 004.

PRENTICE RULE

Named after noted optician Charles Prentice, the formula known as the **Prentice rule** is used to determine the amount of prism, desired or not, which is present in a lens with an established pupillary distance. The formula is prism = (**decentration** × diopters) / 10.

For example, with a +3.00 diopter Rx, the patient's right PD was measured as 31 mm, but after assembly, the right PD in the eyeglasses actually measures at 35 mm. Using the formula, we take the amount of decentration (deviation from the desired PD), which is 4 mm. Multiply 4 × 3 diopters to get 12, then divide by 10 to arrive at 1.2 diopters of prism that has been accidentally induced in this lens.

EXAMPLE 1

Determine the amount of unwanted prism that has been induced in this eyewear: −1.50 sph OU, measured PD was 63, PD on glasses = 57.

In this pair of glasses, the powers are such that there was a reasonable margin of error. Unfortunately, this margin has been exceeded.

Using the Prentice rule, prism = (decentration × diopters) / 10, we can plug in the difference in PD (6 mm) and the lens power, to calculate the unwanted prism as follows: (6 × 1.50) / 10, or 9 / 10, = 0.9 diopters of prism that has been induced. This pair of glasses must be remade.

EXAMPLE 2

Calculate how far off the PD can be in this pair of glasses before it is out of tolerance: OD −1.25 −1.00 X 180, OS −0.50 −1.50 X 090.

This question has two parts: First, we must determine the powers at the 180th meridian. Second, we must reconfigure the Prentice rule to solve for decentration.

The right lens has a cylinder axis of 180; therefore, no cylinder power comes into play at the horizontal. The left lens, with its axis of 90, causes all of the cylinder power to be effective at the horizontal, making the powers at 180 OD −1.25, OS −2.00.

If we assume the maximum tolerable horizontal prism for each eye to be 0.33 diopters, we can then use the inverted Prentice rule as follows: OD (0.33 × 10) / 1.25 = 2.64 mm of tolerable decentration, OS (0.33 × 10) / 2.00 = 1.65 mm of tolerable decentration.

Example 3

Determine the amount of vertical imbalance that has been induced in this pair of glasses:

OD +2.00 sph, OS +2.75 sph, OD centers 3 mm higher than OS.

Because vertical imbalance is relative, this is a case where it is imperative to pay attention to which lens has the stronger power. The vertical imbalance will be read at the weaker of the two.

With the weaker OD lens, applying the Prentice rule gives us (3 mm × 2.00 diopters) / 10 = 0.6 diopters of vertical imbalance. This pair of glasses, or at least whichever lens has the displaced OC, must be remade.

Example 4

Calculate how far one OC can be above or below the other in the following prescription:

−1.50 −2.00 X 091, −0.75 −3.00 X 46.

This question has two parts. First, we must determine the effective powers at the 90th meridian for each lens. Second, we must invert the Prentice rule to solve for decentration, to determine the maximum allowable vertical displacement in the lens that has the weaker power at 90.

Because the OD lens has an axis of nearly 90 degrees, we can disregard the cylinder power completely in the 90th meridian. The OS lens, however, will have roughly 50% of the cylinder power in play at 90. Therefore, whereas at first glance the left lens might appear to be weaker, the effective vertical powers are just the opposite. The left lens reveals itself to be −2.25 in the 90th, and we will concentrate on the weaker OD lens.

Use the inverted Prentice rule, as follows: (0.33 × 10) / 1.50 = 2.2, which gives a maximum of 2.2 mm that the right OC can be vertically displaced from the left, before this pair of glasses fails inspection.

Determining the Dioptric Power of a Lens Given a Focal Length

Example 1

Determine the dioptric power of a lens, given a focal length of 200 mm.

The relationship of focal length to dioptric power is reciprocal. This means that the power of a lens is equal to 1 divided by the focal length. In this formula, focal length is expressed in meters.

First, we would need to convert millimeters into meters, which in this case equals 0.2 meters. Using the focal length formula, 1 divided by 0.2 gives us 5, meaning the lens in question will have 5.00 diopters of power.

EXAMPLE 2

Calculate the focal length of an 8.00 D lens.

Because the relationship of focal length to dioptric power is reciprocal, the formula can be reversed at will. The dioptric power of a lens is equal to 1 divided by its focal length, and, conversely, the focal length is equal to 1 divided by its power.

Approaching this problem from the latter direction, we can easily calculate 1 divided by 8 to reach 0.125, meaning that this lens will have a focal length of 125 mm.

DETERMINING AMOUNT AND DIRECTION OF CHANGE IN EFFECTIVE POWER

EXAMPLE 1

Determine the amount and direction of change in effective power for a −9.00 D lens refracted at a 15 mm vertex but fitted at 11 mm.

The formula for this is as follows: $Dc = D / (1 - dD)$, where D is the written power, d is the vertex deviation in meters, and Dc is the resulting change in effective power. The final direction of the change will depend on whether the lens is plus or minus.

Inserting the numbers from this example, we get $Dc = 9 / (1 - [0.004 \times 9])$, or $9 / (1 - 0.036)$, or $9 / 0.964$, giving an answer of 9.34. Because this is a minus lens, which always increases in effective power with a closer vertex distance, 9.34 D is the effective power at that new distance. (A plus lens of equal strength would change in the opposite direction, downward to 8.66 D.)

EXAMPLE 2

Calculate the compensated power that should be ordered to accommodate a +12.00 lens fitted 5 mm closer to the eye than during the refraction.

In this example, we must first determine the change in effective power at the new vertex distance and then we determine which direction it ends up in.

The formula is *Dc* = *D* / (1 – *dD*). From our example, we can insert 12 for *D* and 0.005 for *d*, giving us 12 / (1 – [0.005 × 12]), or 12 / (1 – 0.06), or 12 / 0.94, giving a result of 12.77. Because the lens is plus, this means that the effective power at that distance will be 0.77 less, or 11.23 D. Thus, 12.77 D is the actual lens that should be ordered to compensate for the loss in effective power.

Fresnel's Formula

Fresnel's formula (named for the famed 19th-century French physicist Augustin-Jean Fresnel) is used to determine the total amount of light reflected from a single optical surface of a given refractive index. This decimal value is known as reflectance. It must be multiplied by 2, to account for both surfaces of a lens, each of which reflects away some light. To express the decimal result as a percentage, it can be multiplied by 100.

Example

Calculate the reflectance of a 1.74 index lens.

The formula is *R* = ([*n*–1] / [*n*+1]) squared, where *R* is the reflectance and *n* is the refractive index. In our example, ([1.74 – 1] / [1.74 + 1]) squared = (0.74 / 2.74) squared = 0.27 squared = 0.0729 per lens surface. Multiply this by 2 for a total of 0.1458 for both sides of a clear lens. This means that of the light attempting to pass through a 1.74 index lens, 14.58% is being reflected away.

Invention of the First Multifocal Lens

None other than Benjamin Franklin is credited with creating the first bifocal lens known to man. He had grown tired of switching between his regular glasses and the ones he used for reading, and so he carefully cut the lenses from each of them in half, horizontally, and pieced the top half of his distance lenses and the bottom half of his reading lenses into the same frame. There are some accounts that indicate that European opticians may have stumbled upon this idea at around the same time. However, this basic design became the standard form of bifocal lenses for decades to come and can still be found under the names executive, full-segment, or even Ben Franklin bifocals, although they are now molded as a single piece with two distinct front curvatures.

The later development of the trifocal lens also employed this design, at first. In this case, the front of the lens would have three distinct curvatures, rather than two, producing a distance power at the top, a reading power at the bottom, and an intermediate power in a central strip about 7–10 mm tall.

Structure of a Segmented Bifocal or Trifocal

A **segmented bifocal** was an improvement over the initial double-curvature bifocal designs, which often required an extremely thick lens and troublesome frame insertion. This design used what appears as a tiny piece (or segment) of a plus lens equal to the add power overlaid on a single front curvature, positioned below the center and toward the nose. These segments have appeared in a variety of shapes, the oldest being completely circular spots (still available as a round-segment or **Kryptok** bifocal) and the newer ones with the top of the circle truncated (known as a **flat-top bifocal**). The latter design was expanded on, adding a small ribbon of slightly flatter curvature on top of the truncated reading add, to create a flat-top trifocal.

Note that the basic design above (with the lens blanks soon being manufactured as a single piece) assumes that a homogeneous material is used to make the lens. The same effect, however, could be obtained by inlaying a small piece of a denser material, enabling the segment to sit flush with the front surface. This fused approach became common in the form of crown glass lenses with inlaid segments of flint glass. However, the practice was never pursued beyond glass.

No-Line Multifocals

The line in bifocal and trifocal lenses was often problematic for patients, due to the **image jump** at the segment line and to the obvious cosmetic concerns. The early 20th century saw several attempts to eliminate the line, resulting in marginally successful designs such as the blended bifocal, some of which have persisted well into modern times. By the early 1970s, this effort led to the first commercially successful **progressive addition lens**, in which the front curvature was gradually steepened toward the bottom of the lens in order to create a progressively stronger add power below the optical center.

These lenses use an aspheric front curvature to produce the central variable-add section, while dissipating the remaining curvature differences to either side. Early versions of these lenses were somewhat crude in their approach, producing enormous areas of distortion to either side of the **add corridor**. More recent research and development, coupled with improvements in manufacturing, have produced designs that have minimized these peripheral distortions and maximized the useful corridor.

Multifocal Lenses for Work-Specific Uses

Traditional multifocals provide appropriate correction in visual ranges normally encountered by the average patient. But there are ways in which this correction may be optimized for other purposes, such as an occupation requiring more intermediate-range and less distance vision. Lenses made for such purposes are called occupational multifocals.

One of the most common occupational lenses is the double-D bifocal, which has add segments above and below the line of sight. These are ideal for folks who require up-close vision both high and low, such as an electrician looking up into a service panel or a painter working under an eave. A variation on this theme can be found in executive (or full-segment) designs as well, and the two adds may be ordered in differing powers or as equal to each other.

When people began spending hours at computer screens, the need became apparent for greater amounts of intermediate vision, and so the CRT (for cathode ray tube, the early, boxy monitors) trifocal was born. It had an intermediate ribbon of 14 mm high, twice the norm. More recently, we have been seeing task-specific progressive lens styles that address the same problem, maximizing the intermediate zone at the expense of distance and near or doing away with distance vision altogether.

Archaic and Seldom-Seen Multifocal Styles

Intended as a compromise between the small size of a round-segment bifocal and the bulkiness of the full-segment, the Ultex bifocal enjoyed a brief period of popularity. This lens featured a large reading area with a semicircular shape, bonded across most of the bottom edge of the lens.

The **curve-top bifocal** was once considered fashionable. This was a variation on the flat-top bifocal, with the top of the segment having a gentle upward curvature rather than being straight across.

The **oval-segment bifocal** was once briefly popular, but its tiny size limited its appeal. It became more commonly seen on high-plus aspherics, where its small size and odd shape were more at home.

A precursor to progressive lenses was the **blended bifocal**. This lens featured a round reading area, resembling a round-segment with its edges blended away. This style is still available today, although it has very limited appeal due to the large distortion ring around the usable add power.

An odd marriage of flat-top and progressive, the **Smart Seg** was never very popular. This lens looked like a flat-top bifocal, but the reading area contained a seamless intermediate-to-near progression.

Common Standard Lens Materials

For centuries, the only material acceptable for optical lenses of any kind was glass. It was rigid enough to hold a complex shape, and it could be made perfectly clear. Until the mid-20th century, no material was considered the equal of **crown glass**. (Flint glass did achieve some use as a thinner alternative for high prescriptions, for inlaid multifocal segments, and in some telescope optics.)

With the advent of plastics, manufacturers began experimenting with lenses made of acrylic and other polymers. But it was not until the mid-1970s that a truly viable alternative to glass was born. During the design phase of the *Space Shuttle Columbia*, a polymer was sought that would make a suitable lens for the gauges in the shuttle cockpit. The 39th material in those experiments was the winner, which was designated as Columbia Resin #39, or **CR-39**. This material was of good enough optical quality to rival glass, and it quickly took the optical industry by storm, edging out glass as the new default lens material of choice.

Common Standard Lens Materials Requiring High Shatter Resistance

During the 1970s, one of the materials explored for use in optical lenses was polycarbonate. Polycarbonate had been used in industrial applications since the 1950s, but with improvements to the refining processes in its manufacture, something like optical quality became possible. The material quickly gained acceptance for sport and safety applications, due to its highly shatter-resistant nature. (Polycarbonate is 60 times more impact resistant than glass.) It is also lighter weight and thinner than glass or plastic lenses, with a refractive index of 1.58, although it is of somewhat lower optical quality than either.

Around the turn of this century, a material called **Trivex**, initially developed for military use, became available as an optical lens material. This offered a similar impact resistance to that of polycarbonate, along with a similar weight, while boasting optical clarity equal to that of glass. Its primary drawback is that its refractive index is a mere 1.53, nearly the same as glass. That and its relative expense make it a less desirable alternative for higher prescriptions, although it still has uses where safety and optical clarity are the primary concerns.

Thinner and Lighter Lens Materials

When a patient's prescription would result in an undesirably thick lens, a lens material with a higher refractive index than glass or plastic (nominally 1.5) is often recommended. The first **high-index lenses** to come into common use had an index of 1.56, substantially reducing lens thicknesses. But this material was quickly outshone when lenses were introduced in 1.60 index and above, relegating 1.56 to the term **mid-index**. Then 1.60 in turn was overshadowed by 1.67 index, which was then overshadowed by 1.70 and 1.74. The higher the index, the thinner the resulting lens. These lenses are all made of variations in polyurethanes, and most are commonly referred to as **thin & light lenses**.

The drawback to these lenses is that they each offer reduced optical clarity as a trade-off to thinness. As the index increases, so does the **chromatic aberration** and the **reflectivity**, whereas the Abbe value goes sharply downward. In addition, the cost of these lenses generally increases with the index. These considerations limit their recommended use to patients with the strongest prescriptions, where the weight and thickness of the lenses become of primary concern.

Variable-Tint Lenses

Lenses that are made to alter their color with varying lighting conditions are known collectively as **photochromatic lenses**. These are not actual lens materials; rather, they are treatments applied during manufacturing. Thus, many different lens materials and styles may be available as photochromatic lenses.

The first photochromatic lenses were glass lenses, and they were called PhotoGray. The crown glass was impregnated during the manufacturing process with silver halide crystals, which darkened when struck by light. There was also a PhotoBrown version, as well as a PhotoSun variant that began with a 50% tint and got extremely dark in sunlight.

Newer lenses, in plastics, polycarbonates, and polyurethanes, are treated with an imbibing process, wherein the lens absorbs the photochromatic agent. These lenses go by trade names such as Transitions and SunSensors, but they do essentially the same thing as their glass forbears, darkening in sunlight.

These lenses all have uses in cases where a patient is in and out of doors a lot and can't be taking the time to switch eyewear. They do not equal the sun protection of a dedicated pair of sunglasses, but for those looking for increased visual comfort in a single pair of eyeglasses, photochromatics can fill the need.

Prism

In its simplest form, a prism is a triangular wedge of light-transmitting material. The widest point of the prism is called its **base**, whereas the narrowest point is called the **apex**. Light passing through the prism is refracted toward the base of the prism, which results in shifting the optical image in the opposite direction, toward the apex.

A prism as it fits into the overall scheme of a prescription lens is a bit more complicated. It may help to think of a plus lens as essentially two prisms base to base; conversely, a minus lens is two prisms apex to apex. Thus, a plus lens with prism in the prescription would result in the two bases meeting at a point away from the center, whereas in a minus lens, the apexes would meet somewhere off-center. With this in mind, it is easy to see how a desired prism might be induced simply by repositioning the center of the lens. (The greater the overall lens power, the easier this is to do.)

Common Uses for Prescribed Prism

Prism may be prescribed for various reasons. In cases in which the eyes have mild difficulty working together or doing so causes eyestrain, mild prism is often used **palliatively**, in order to help the eyes relax while they do their job. When **diplopia** (double vision) is present, prism may be used correctively to shift one or both eyes' image enough to merge with the other, restoring normal binocular vision. Prism can also be used in cases in which a portion of the visual field has been lost (for example, due to injury or a stroke), positioned so as to shift the entire remaining field of vision, restoring some lost peripheral perception.

Inducing Prescribed Prism by Decentering a Single-Vision Lens

The power of a lens will determine how much prism is induced by decentering it. Just as this can induce an error, it can sometimes be put to work for the optician to produce a desired prismatic effect.

If a lens has a power of −4.00 D and we wish to induce 2 diopters of prism base in, this is a simple matter. By inverting the Prentice formula to solve for the decentration, we can insert the known values as follows: (2 prism diopters × 10) divided by a 4 diopter lens, or 20 divided by 4, gives us the 5 mm of decentration necessary to do the job. Because this is a minus lens and because moving the OC away from the nose will increase the base-in prism, we know that the 5 mm decentration will be outward.

If, on the other hand, the lens has a power of +1.00 and we wish to induce 4 diopters of prism, it probably cannot be done. In this case, (4 prism diopters × 10) divided by 1 gives us 40 mm of decentration to induce that much prism in such a low-power lens, which would likely cause the lens not to cut out.

Amount and Direction of Decentration Needed to Induce a 5.00 D BI Prism in a −3.00 D Lens

The amount of decentration necessary can be determined by inverting the Prentice formula, as follows: decentration = (prism × 10) / diopters. Plugging in the numbers, we get (5 × 10) / 3, or 50/3, which gives us the 16.67 mm of decentration necessary.

Although this might seem like a large number, it may be doable. Being a minus lens, base-in prism will be induced by moving the OC away from the bridge (thickening the nasal edge), which is counter to the usual inward-decentering to match the PD, and it therefore works in our favor. If the lens would normally have to be moved inward 6 mm for the sake of the PD, and the prism calls for 16 in the other direction, then we are looking at a net outward decentering of only 10 mm. If, on the other hand, this were a +3.00 lens, we would be looking at a total inward movement of 22 mm, which would probably keep the lens from cutting out.

Ways in Which Prism in Eyewear Can Be Detrimental

Whenever prism is present in a lens that did not call for it, it is called unwanted prism error. It is generally undesirable, and it may render the lens in question unacceptable. Dispensing eyewear with prism error to a patient can result in headaches, disorientation, or in severe cases, diplopia, or double vision.

The amount of prism present can be determined using the Prentice rule, or it can be read on a lensometer. In either event, it is measured by defining the optical center's deviation from an established reference point, either some premarked reference point or the patient's PD. When the error is in a vertical direction, no more than one-third diopter is acceptable. When the error is horizontal, a total of two-thirds diopter is allowable.

Ocular Anatomy, Physiology, and Pathology

Anterior and Posterior Segments of the Eye

The eye consists of many elements, but it can roughly be divided into the **anterior segment** and the **posterior segment**. The anterior segment consists of the cornea, iris, pupil, and lens, whereas the posterior segment encompasses the large chamber behind the lens, the retina, and the eye's interface with the optic nerve.

The anterior segment can be further subdivided into the anterior chamber, which is behind the cornea but in front of the iris, and the smaller posterior chamber, which lies between the iris and the lens. Both chambers are filled with the **aqueous humor**, a watery material that is responsible for holding the **intraocular pressure**.

The posterior segment of the eye is filled with a thicker substance called the **vitreous humor**, which helps the eyeball maintain its shape. It is loosely bonded with the nervous tissue lining the rear of the eyeball, called the **retina**. The vitreous humor can become clouded over time, because its quality deteriorates with age.

Retina

The purpose of the retina is to gather light that it receives and transmit the light to the brain for interpretation as an image. It lies along the inside posterior surface of the eye, as part of a multilayered structure known collectively as the **neural tunic**.

The primary tissue of the retina is composed of millions of specialized light-receptor cells called **rods** and **cones**. The rods are highly sensitive to lower levels of light but can only perceive in black and white. The cones are responsible for color perception, but they require brighter light in order to function. The greatest concentration of rods and cones is found in the macula, which is the central area of the retina, and especially at the fovea, which is at the center of the macula; thus, this area provides the most detailed visual images.

The retina is connected at a spot below the macula to the **optic nerve**, which transmits the image data to the brain. The point at which the optic nerve joins the retina (the **optic disk**, or optic nerve head) has neither rods nor cones, and so this point represents a small blind spot in the normal visual field.

Refraction of Light in the Normal Eye

The **cornea** and the **crystalline lens** of the eye work together to bring light to a focus at the rear of the eye, much like the objective and eyepiece of a telescope.

The cornea is the primary refractive body of the eye, with a typical refractive index of 1.37 and a power of around +43.00 diopters. In the healthy eye, its shape (and power) is fixed and does not change. The crystalline lens, on the other hand, is made to alter its shape to adapt for changing focal needs. This gives the normal eye the ability to focus on nearby objects as well as those far away, a process known as **accommodation**. The lens has an average index of about 1.39 (higher in the center and lower at the edges) and a refracting power of anywhere from +14.00 to +19.00 diopters.

Cornea

The cornea is separate from the vascular elements of the eye and the rest of the body. It obtains all of its oxygen directly from the air.

The cornea consists of several layers of specialized tissue, the outermost being the **epithelium**, which is a tough, protective covering. The innermost layer, facing the iris, is called the **endothelium**. The bulk of the cornea, roughly 90% of its thickness, is between those two and is called the stroma. On either side of the **stroma**, a thin membrane forms a boundary to the outer layers, Bowman's membrane just under the epithelium and Descemet's membrane against the endothelium.

Physical Changes in Normal Eye's Refractive Ability as Patient Ages

In a normal, youthful eye, the crystalline lens is squeezed and stretched by the **ciliary body**, a network of tiny muscles that surround the lens. Squeezing the lens causes it to thicken, providing more plus power to focus on near objects.

As the eye ages, the lens gets stiffer and is no longer able to change its shape nearly as much. This means that although the eye may retain perfect vision at infinity (anything more than 20 feet away), continuing to bring light from those distances into focus, it will lose its ability to focus on objects within the first few feet of the patient, without the extra help of reading lenses or bifocals. This is a progressive condition (known as presbyopia) that affects all patients at some age, and it is not presently correctable by any surgical procedure.

Common Surgical Means of Improving Vision

The first refractive surgeries, such as **radial keratotomy**, involved making a series of small incisions in the outer surface of the cornea. This caused the shape of the cornea to slump, changing its refractive power. The results were mixed, and the resulting vision was frequently unstable. Newer procedures involved using a laser to actively sculpt the cornea's curvature. These are called **photorefractive keratectomy** (PRK) and laser-assisted in-situ keratomileusis (**LASIK**). The major difference between the two is that in LASIK, a flap of endothelial tissue is first lifted up, allowing the sculpted area to be covered back up afterward for easier healing. Results from PRK and LASIK are generally more acceptable, but all of these procedures are irreversible.

In extreme cases, the vision can be improved by implanting an **intraocular lens** just in front of the eye's crystalline lens. This procedure, though technically reversible, is usually avoided because of the high risks always associated with invasive eye surgery. There have also been attempts to develop implantable devices that would act as corneal shims (under the name InTacts, among others) resting just under the epithelium to alter the corneal profile. These are less invasive and are fully reversible, but so far they have only been approved for very minor refractive errors.

Eyelid

The eyelids act in several ways to keep the eyes healthy. The most obvious is their ability to keep the eye moist. Blinking is a near-autonomic action, much like breathing — a person may stop breathing for a few moments, but eventually the nervous system takes over. With each blink, the lids bathe the surface of the eyes with fresh tears. You may briefly force yourself to stop blinking, but eventually the lids will blink, keeping the eyes moistened.

In addition, the lids help prevent foreign matter from entering the eye. If an object approaches the face rapidly, or if the eyes sense that you are about to encounter dirt or dust, the lids close in a protective blink reflex, keeping the danger away from the eyes' sensitive surface.

The upper and lower eyelids meet at the **canthus**, commonly called the corner of the eye. The side toward the nose is called the medial canthus, whereas the opposite one is called the lateral canthus.

Tear Production

The tears come from a variety of sources around the eye, but the majority of tear production takes place in the **lacrimal glands**, located just above and behind the upper eyelids. In addition, the tear film is augmented by secretions from the **meibomian glands** (located along the inside edges of the lids) and from the **lacrimal caruncle**, located near the medial canthus, the nasal corners of the eyes.

The tear layer is spread across the eye with each blink. Excess tears are siphoned away by the lacrimal puncta (also located near the medial canthus), down into the lacrimal sac and eventually into the nasal cavity.

Eye Movement

The motion of the eye is controlled by a system of six muscles attached just behind the eyelids. There are two muscles above, two below, and one to each side. Muscles above the eye are referred to as superior, those below are called inferior, and the ones to each side are lateral and medial, with medial being on the side toward the nose. Muscles known as **rectus** move the eye in one direction, by pulling it horizontally or vertically, whereas oblique muscles allow the eye to roll in more complex directions.

The superior rectus, for example, pulls the eye straight back, to look upward, whereas the inferior rectus turns the eye downward. The medial rectus causes the eye to turn toward the nose, whereas the lateral rectus turns it toward the temple. The superior oblique helps the eye roll down and to the side, whereas the inferior oblique rolls it up and to the side.

Emmetropia

When a patient's vision has no defects, the images come to a focus evenly on the retina with no distortion, and he reads at 20/20 on the Snellen chart, he is said to have the enviable condition of emmetropia (from the Greek word emmetros, meaning well proportioned). This condition has no diagnosis code, for the simple reason that it represents a diagnosis of nothing.

Many people with mild refractive errors go undiagnosed, simply because their vision is good enough to satisfy them and does not interfere with their daily activity. This is not the same as emmetropia, which can only be determined by an eye exam.

Nearsightedness and Farsightedness

The normal function of the refractive elements of the eye is to bring light to a sharp focus at the back of the eye, on the retina. This may fail because of the eye being too long or too short, the lens and cornea having too little or too much power, or some combination of both.

For whatever reason, when light comes to a focus before reaching the retina, a person is said to be myopic, or nearsighted. When the light comes to a focus at a point that would theoretically be behind the retina, a person is hyperopic, or farsighted.

Astigmatism

When the rays of light do not all reach the retina together, with some coming to focus behind or in front of the retina, the condition is called **astigmatism**. It is caused by an asphericity of the cornea or the lens, resulting in more than one curvature refracting light in two different ways.

This condition may appear with or without underlying myopia or hyperopia. When an eye focuses some of the light on the retina but some in front of it, the condition is called simple myopic astigmatism (for example, plano −1.00 X 90). When some of the light is in focus at the retina but some behind it, we call it simple hyperopic astigmatism (plano +1.00 X 90, or +1.00 −1.00 X 180). When an eye is already myopic or hyperopic, the condition is called compound myopic or hyperopic astigmatism (−2.00 −1.00 X 90, or +2.00 −1.00 X 90). In cases in which the astigmatism causes some of the light to focus in front of the retina and some behind, it is called mixed astigmatism (+1.00 −2.00 X 90).

Presbyopia

The aging eye steadily loses its ability to accommodate, or refocus, between distant and near objects. This is a result of the eye's crystalline lens declining in elasticity. The eye will bring light reflected from faraway objects to a focus on the retina, but it becomes unable to focus on closer objects. This refractive error is known as **presbyopia**, and it is an accepted facet of aging. It is generally not considered a refractive error until it begins to impact normal day-to-day function, which normally happens in a patient's mid-40s.

Diplopia

Although not technically a refractive error, this condition, known as **diplopia**, deserves discussion here. Diplopia is when the eyes are producing images that do not line up with each other, either due to a muscular imbalance in the eyes, a condition of the central nervous system, or a head injury. But unlike most other pathological conditions, this one is often corrected optically, just as a refractive error would be.

In this case, for whatever reason, the light is focusing properly on the retina, but either the resulting images are too different to fuse into one or the information is being misinterpreted by the optic nerve or the brain. In the former case, the problem is addressed by shifting the incoming light to one side, enough to draw the eyes into a better position for **binocular fusion** to occur. In the latter, it may be a matter of simply moving the focal point to a slightly different area of the retina, to fool the brain into seeing objects in the same location with both eyes.

Eye Conditions Where the Two Eyes Do Not Function Together Naturally

In **amblyopia** (wandering eye), the optician may be called upon to be an active participant in the patient's treatment. Prism is often applied in such cases. This might be ground in, or it might be applied as a **Fresnel** or press-on prism, which is cut into shape from a sheet of static-cling vinyl. Just as with ground-in prism, strict attention must be paid to the strength and direction of the prism. Eye conditions resulting in a tendency for the eye to wander are called **phorias**. **Esophoria** is a tendency for the eye to wander inward, whereas **exophoria** would be outward wandering.

In mild amblyopic cases with little or no diplopia, the doctor may order an **occlusion film**, cut and applied in the same manner over the stronger eye, in order to force the weaker one to work harder. (Sometimes, an eye patch is used instead.)

Amblyopia's cousin **strabismus** (crossed eyes) will always require prism, if not surgical intervention. Eye conditions resulting in these definite turnings of the eye are called **tropias**. **Esotropia** is an inward turning, whereas **exotropia** would be outward turning.

Slab-Off Lens

In monocular aphakia (absence of a lens) or extreme **anisometropia** (a large power difference between the eyes), a presbyopic patient may have trouble combining images at the reading level, due to the large amount of vertical prism induced that far from the optical center. This may be corrected by use of a **slab-off lens**, which uses bicentric grinding to produce base-up prism in the bottom portion of the lens with the most minus or least plus power.

The amount of slab-off needed can be calculated using the Prentice formula, given a known **reading level**. This is the distance that the eye drops from the optical center in order to use the reading area of the lens, and by default it is usually assumed to be about 10 mm. Thus, if the distance correction in the OD lens is +1.50 and the OS lens is −7.50, the formula is applied using the 9-diopter difference, as follows: $9D \times 10$ mm / 10 = 9 diopters of prism induced at the reading level in the left eye. Because this is a minus lens, the induced prism will be base-down and it will be corrected by slab-off prism of $9D$ base-up. (Plus-power lenses will use **reverse slab**, a special lens blank, in the exact opposite manner.)

EXAMPLE 1

Calculate the amount and location of slab-off prism needed for an anisometropic presbyope with the following prescription:

OD +0.50, OS −6.00, add +2.50.

The patient with a prescription such as this will probably find it impossible to read without some form of prism compensation at the reading level. His left lens will be producing base-down prism at that point, whereas his right lens will be doing the opposite. Base-up prism in the lower half of his left lens will solve the problem.

To determine just how much, use the Prentice formula: Prism = (decentration × diopters) / 10. In this case, decentration is the 10 mm that his eye drops in order to read through the bifocal and diopters refers to the difference between the two lenses, which amounts to 6.50. So, (10 × 6.5) / 10 = 6.50 D of slab-off prism that should be applied to the left lens.

EXAMPLE 2

Calculate the amount and location of slab prism needed for a monocular aphakic presbyope with the following prescription:

OD +1.25, OS +14.50, add +2.25.

The aphakic patient (no crystalline lens) will have an extremely high-plus lens prescribed for the aphakic eye. Therefore, there may be no lens of sufficient minus power to support bicentric grinding for a slab-off configuration. In this case, the optician will have to use a reverse-slab lens on the left side.

The choice of prism powers in the reverse-slab blank may be limited, and so the closest possible value will have to be selected. But the initial calculations are the same, using the Prentice formula: Prism = (decentration × diopters) / 10. In our example, the diopters is the power difference, which is 13.25, and the reading level is the 10 mm decentration. So, (10 × 13.25) / 10 equals 13.25 diopters of reverse slab.

Ptosis

When a patient has an eyelid that droops enough to obscure the vision, the condition is called **ptosis**. This can be caused by inflammation from an eye infection, as a side-effect of eye surgery, or a number of other causes.

Although most modern ophthalmologists will often correct this condition with a surgical procedure known as a **blepharectomy**, there are still situations in which surgery is contraindicated. In these cases, the optician may be called upon to use a **ptosis crutch** to correct the problem. This is a small prop that is attached to the rear of the patient's frame, and precisely positioned so as to lift the eyelid out of the patient's line of sight. Needless to say, these should be used with extreme caution.

Acute Medical Conditions of the Eye

The optician can sometimes be the professional who first catches a new or developing problem for the patient, simply because he may be the first person the patient happens to mention it to. Sometimes this can help avert a disaster.

Retinal detachment is a condition in which the retinal tissue tears loose and begins to slump forward within the eye. The patient will usually notice a large amount of flashes and floaters in his vision, followed by part of the visual field going black. This is a medical emergency and can result in blindness if not treated immediately.

Glaucoma is a condition that causes runaway intraocular pressure. The patient may complain of severe pain in one eye or a severe headache centered around the eye. If left unchecked, the patient's visual field will narrow to a spot. This also requires immediate treatment.

Review Video: What is the Difference Between Glaucoma and Cataracts?
Visit mometrix.com/academy and enter code: 279024

Any sudden visual disturbance should raise red flags in the optician's mind. An unchecked diabetic, for example, may have wild fluctuations in visual acuity. Left untreated, his condition may lead to retinopathy or even blindness. The use of adjustable-power glasses may help such patients until they are stabilized.

Less Acute Ocular Pathologies

There are many conditions the optician cannot help, but knowing about them may improve the general quality of the patient's care. **Keratoconus** (literally, cone-shaped cornea) is when the cornea bulges outward excessively. Whereas some of these patients may be treated by wearing rigid contact lenses to mold the cornea into a better shape, many are never able to adapt and must be optically best-corrected with glasses. These patients will have high amounts of mixed astigmatism at oblique axes (such as +2.50 −6.00 X 47), and their prescriptions may change frequently. Aphakia is much less common today, but if a patient is not able to have an intraocular lens implant for some reason, he may be left in this condition, in which one eye requires a very high plus lens (+12.00 D or greater). If the condition is monocular, the patient will suffer from **aniseikonia** (unequal sizes of the retinal images) and image swim. If binocular, the patient will have reduced peripheral vision, as well as very heavy glasses. **Graves' disease** is a thyroid condition with a characteristic symptom of protruding eyes. These patients will often require unusual compound prism corrections, which they can expect to shift radically once or twice a year.

Ophthalmic Products

Metal Frame Materials

Many metallic materials have been used for eyeglass frames over the years. Gold and silver were once common, although their cost probably limited eyeglasses to the more well-to-do patients. Although both were easily worked, they did have a tendency to stretch over time, and their softness made it difficult to hold an adjustment.

Improvements in metal refining and fabrication led to more advanced frame materials such as aluminum being tried. Aluminum was extremely lightweight, but it tended to be brittle. Various metal alloys were experimented with, until a reasonably durable nickel-copper-manganese alloy called **Monel** was developed. It was rigid, held its shape, and was relatively inexpensive. Its drawbacks were that without an outer coating or plating of some kind, Monel would degrade under constant contact with a patient's perspiration or skin acidity and this could produce mild allergic reactions. (Often, a frame would be Monel covered with a gold electroplating.)

More recently, midrange to high-end frames have been made using stainless steel and titanium. Stainless steel is extremely durable and hypoallergenic, but it can make larger frames heavy. Titanium is also hypoallergenic and even more durable, but it is the lightest weight metal of all. It is very expensive and is usually found in high-end frames.

Constructions That Do Not Use a Complete Frame

The two types of eyewear using less than a full frame fall into two broad categories: **rimless** and **semi-rimless** frames.

In the semi-rimless frame, there is a complete over- or understructure that is continuous from temple to temple. The frame front will usually go above the lens, leaving the bottom edge exposed. The lenses are held in place either by nylon cord stretched around the exposed edge (into a grooved channel cut in the lens edge) or by sharply pointed corners in the edged shape that fit into corresponding notches in the frame front.

A rimless frame has no continuous structure, and generally consists of three pieces joined by the lenses themselves. Typically, either small screws and nuts or a pin-and-bushing configuration will fasten the end pieces and bridge to the lenses. There have also been a handful of frames made with variations on this theme, such as lenses that snap into place.

Most Common Nonmetallic Frame Material

During the mid-20th century, the search for a lightweight, durable, and hypoallergenic material for eyeglasses turned to plastics. A polymer called **cellulose acetate**, previously used to coat airplane wings, became accepted as an ophthalmic material for its abilities to hold a rigid shape, to be easily worked with mild heat, and its hypoallergenic properties. Moreover, it could be made in any color imaginable, and it was very inexpensive to produce. This material is now commonly referred to as **Zyl**, which is short for Zylonite, one of the common trade names under which cellulose acetate was originally manufactured.

Other Nonmetallic Frame Material Options

Various improvements in plastic frame materials have been brought to market over the years, but none very successfully. In the mid-1960s, a slightly lighter weight version of cellulose acetate was developed and patented, under the name Optyl. This material had a memory, in that if distorted, applying heat would return it to its original shape. A huge drawback was in the difficulty of adjusting these frames, which would turn to spaghetti under heat but rapidly go brittle as they cooled, often snapping in an optician's hands.

Other manufacturers attempted to duplicate the shortcomings of Optyl while building on its strengths. These materials are marketed under trade names such as SPX and Grilamid, and they produce very thin and lightweight frames. They are easier to adjust, but they have none of the memory ability known to Optyl and are easily overshrunk when heated a little too much.

Nylon frames were popular for several years but never achieved lasting market share. They produced a lightweight frame with some flexibility, but they tended to get brittle with age unless routinely soaked in water. Today, they are rarely seen except in certain sport and safety applications.

Common Types of Lens Recommended for a Patients Younger Than Age 40

The typical patient younger than age 40 suffers from myopia, hyperopia, astigmatism, or some combination of these. In all cases, this is corrected by the use of a **single-vision lens**, which typically has one curvature on its front and one or two on its back side. Its job is simply to correct the basic refractive error, producing a sharp focal point at the retina and counteracting the visual deficit often found in children and young adults.

Single-vision lenses can also be prescribed as near-vision-only glasses for patients in their mid-40s and over. In this case, they are for intermittent use, correcting the visual deficit of an otherwise emmetropic patient whose eyes are simply no longer able to focus on near objects.

Common Types of Lenses Used for a Patient Age 40–45 and Above

When the eye can no longer change focus from far to near objects, a lens with more than one sphere power is called for. This is called a **multifocal** lens.

Multifocals come in a wide variety of designs, from the old executive or full-segment style (with two completely separate curvatures), to segmented styles such as the flat-top 28 bifocal, to line-free lenses such as the **progressive-addition lens**.

Progressive lenses have become very popular for two primary reasons. For one, they provide a continuous power change from far to near Rx, giving the patient a little something for every viewing distance, without the cumbersome jumping-off point of a line; and for the other, they are much more cosmetically appealing to the patient. As a result, much research and development has been invested in making these lenses better and more natural feeling.

Computer-Driven Manufacturing

For many years, lens processing was tied to the limitations of technology, in that the tools required for it were only available in 1/8-diopter steps. Therefore, the final lens was only accurate to within 1/8 of a diopter. Newer computer-driven manufacturing techniques have made it possible to bypass that tooling limitation by being able to grind and polish the lens in a single step, thus increasing its accuracy to within 1/100th of a diopter. This translates into more accurate visual correction for the patient.

This new manufacturing capability has been extended to include the possibility for complete customization of the patient's Rx, unbounded by limitations of base curvature. One-of-a-kind aspheric and atoric designs can mean an enhanced visual experience for the patient, as well as improved cosmetics.

Differences Between Older and Newer Progressive Lens Designs

The first progressive lenses were essentially manipulations of the front curvature of the lens down through a central corridor, to produce a stronger lens at the bottom in that small spot. The discrepancy between that resulting curvature and the base curvature of the upper lens was simply blended away, leaving large swaths to either side of the visual field an astigmatic mess that had to simply be ignored.

With the advent of digital modeling technology, research and development brought these lenses back to the drawing table, examining how best to optimize the light passing through the lens at each and every point. This has resulted in effective broadening of the corridors and minimizing of the wasteland zones, giving patients a much-improved visual experience.

Special Lens Designs for Specific Circumstances for Middle-Aged and Older Patients

There are many visual situations that are not necessarily within the standard fitting models. A good example is the 50-year-old golfer. He needs sharp distance vision as well as the ability to read the numbers on his putters and drivers. But a traditional bifocal design puts the reading area directly in his way, as he looks down to line up his shot. For him, inverting a bifocal and putting the near vision at the top of the lens will best fit his needs.

Another prime example is the heavy computer user, who spends a good share of his time not needing distance vision at all, but an intermediate range for viewing his monitor. For these patients, a traditional bifocal can be used with the add power halved and added to the distance portion of the lens, or there are any number of specialty progressive-addition styles that can accomplish the same thing without a line.

For the presbyopic patient who works in a visually demanding situation where precise near vision is required above and below the line of sight, there are several so-called **occupational multifocals** available with segments in both places. Often, these can be further customized by selecting two different add powers, to accommodate specific visual needs in each location.

Occupational Lens

Choosing an Occupational Multifocal for a House Painter

A person painting the exterior of a house will have visual needs at varying distances. These will not always be in the usual locations within the visual field. He will need to read paint cans and see his brushes, so he will need near vision. He will also need a good amount of the intermediate range, for when he is painting at arm's length. And of course, he will need crisp distance vision, in order to navigate ladders and other heights.

For this patient, the double-D multifocal is probably the best choice, with an upper add equal to half of the lower add. This will allow him to see well when he is painting under an eave, or around a window. For fine trim work, he will use the lower segment at full near power. And the majority of the lens will be left to unadulterated distance vision.

The progressive lens makes a spectacularly bad choice for this patient, because there is far too little intermediate, and it is in the wrong place. The waviness of the lower half of the lens could also be a hazard, for example, when climbing a ladder.

Choosing an Occupational Lens for a Presbyopic Auto Mechanic

The auto mechanic primarily has two visual needs, distance and near vision, but not in the usual places. She will need to be able to see belts, hoses, and relays under the hood, and she will need to read from a repair manual on occasion. But she will also need to be looking up from the underside of the car to see small parts, grease fittings, and fine adjustment screws.

This patient could benefit from a double-D multifocal with equal upper and lower near-vision adds. This will give her crisp close-in vision whether she is above or below the car. If she is concerned about the intermediate range and doesn't need distance vision during the course of the workday, the distance portion of the lens could be calculated to provide intermediate vision instead, with the remainder of the add power at the segments.

Choosing an Occupational Lens for the Presbyope Working in a Small Office

Small office settings vary widely, so ask enough questions to flesh out all of the needs encountered during the day.

If the patient works at a computer monitor all day, the intermediate correction is paramount. However, it is rare for this patient never to need to refer to the keyboard, or his phone, or some written material, so you will also need to correct for near. If he can sacrifice distance vision, the entire upper half of the lens can be made as intermediate, and even a simple flat-top bifocal will do. If he thinks he will find the bifocal line too distracting (or cosmetically unappealing), there are any number of progressive-style lenses to do the very same thing.

If the distance vision is important enough to keep, there are variations in the progressive-style occupationals that include a sliver of distance at the very top, but this will infringe upon the intermediate somewhat, and the patient should be made aware.

If the patient works on a small enough monitor, doesn't mind the lines, and wants to keep his distance vision intact, the older 14×35 CRT trifocal is still available and is still a good option.

Current Standard in Lens Materials

For centuries, the glass lens was the gold standard for opticians everywhere because of its superb clarity and stability as a refractive medium. Its major drawbacks were its brittleness and its weight.

Since the mid-1970s, glass has overwhelmingly become supplanted by CR-39, a polymer resin that was literally a by-product of the space age. Half the weight of glass (it was initially marketed during the late 1970s and 1980s as HalfWeight lenses) but with nearly the same optical clarity, this material — often simply referred to as plastic — quickly unseated crown glass as the standard lens material of choice. It was not nearly as brittle as glass, easier to work, and did not require special hardening procedures prior to dispensing. Due to its optical superiority, though, glass has remained in use for small-instrument lenses, optometric refracting equipment, and demanding telescope optics.

Alternative Lens Materials

Although plastic (CR-39) lenses offered several advantages over glass, they are not always the optimal material. Fortunately, we now have several to choose from. Everything other than glass is often categorized as plastic, but there are huge differences between the alternatives.

The first material usually offered in place of CR-39 is polycarbonate, which is extremely tough, lightweight, and has a higher index of refraction. This makes it a good default choice for mildly myopic patients who need thinner and lighter lenses, as well as any situation requiring extra attention to safety, such as children's eyewear, industrial safety applications, and monocular patients. It also works well in drill-mounted eyewear constructions. Trivex offers many of the same advantages, except that its refractive index is lower.

High-index lenses (usually categorized as having a refractive index of 1.60 or higher) are often a good alternative for the highly myopic patient because they can dramatically reduce the thickness and weight in very high prescriptions. Their trade-off is reduced optical clarity.

There are still rare occasions where a crown-glass lens is desirable, such as when a patient must work around caustic chemicals (such as a photographer who develops his own film).

Special Procedures for Dispensing Glass Lenses

Glass lenses, in addition to being a harder-to-work material than any plastics, require very specific hardening techniques prior to dispensing.

One of these is a **heat-tempering** process in a small kiln commonly known as a **Kirk oven**. The lenses are heated to temperatures greater than 1,000°F, and then they are removed and rapidly cooled by air jets from above and below. This results in a particular stress pattern within the lens that prevents it from breaking into dangerous shards, but rather into small, granular chunks that are less likely to cause injury.

The other type of hardening process is called **chemtempering**, and it involves a chemical bath in which the lenses must be soaked for 16 hours.

Both hardening processes are carried out after the lens has been edged and safety beveled, and no further changes can be made after the tempering is complete, because they would alter the stress patterns within the lens and affect its hardness. In addition, each hardened lens must be verified in a **drop-ball tester**, which uses a 5/8-inch steel ball dropped from a height of 50 inches onto the front surface of the lens ... an obvious pass/fail test.

Drawbacks That Influence Choice of Lens Material

No one lens material is perfect for all situations, and each one has its drawbacks. These must be balanced against a variety of factors.

Glass lenses will always provide the very best optics. However, they are heavy, hard to work, brittle, and dangerous in many situations.

CR-39 lenses are lighter weight than glass and are almost identical optically, but they are far from unbreakable, and unlike tempered glass, will shatter into dangerous shards. They also admit around 50% of the ultraviolet light striking them, which is unique among lens materials.

Polycarbonate is very lightweight and nearly indestructible, but it suffers from some of the poorest optical clarity of any material. Equally indestructible Trivex has excellent optics but is not nearly as thin a material as polycarbonate, and it is much more expensive.

High-index lenses offer the thinnest lens profiles of any material, but as the refractive index climbs, the Abbe value, or optical clarity, decreases. The Abbe value of a 1.74 lens is nearly as low as that of polycarbonate.

Lenses That Change Color

There are several variations on photochromatic lenses, meaning lenses that alter their color when struck by light. The earliest such lenses were glass, usually marketed under the name PhotoGray. There was also a PhotoBrown variant, as well as a PhotoSun. The first two would start with about a 10%–15% shade and sun darken to about 60%. The PhotoSun lens began at about 50% and darkened to 80%. In all cases, the color change was brought about by silver halide crystals embedded in the glass during manufacture.

Newer plastic materials used various **imbibing** techniques (soaking the lenses in a chemical bath as the final step in manufacturing) to produce a similar effect and have been sold under names such as Transitions, SunSensors, and InstaShades. Results have been mixed but have generally improved over time. Like their glass ancestors, plastic photochromatics now come in variations like Transitions Brown (self-explanatory) and Transitions XTRActive (which mimics the old PhotoSun). DriveWear is another variation on the latter, not only darkening but changing to an optimal hue for contrast enhancement and reduced eye fatigue.

Most lens types will have some availability in photochromatic options. The number of options will generally correspond to the popularity of the lens design.

Lens with Fixed Color

Originally, if a lens with a fixed tint was desired, it had to be manufactured that way. While in a molten state, the glass was impregnated with a specific material designed to produce a particular color. Obviously, this made for a very limited palate, because only certain colors could be made available and only in predetermined shades. The more commonly used colors acquired names such as Crux-Lite, AOLITE, and so forth. G-15, one of those early colors, persists today in certain sunglass lenses, often still made in glass.

A more common method of producing a colored lens today involves immersing it into a tank of molecular catalytic dye, heated to around 200°F. This has the advantage of allowing almost any color or shade that the patient desires, as well as the ability to apply it to an already-manufactured lens. Nearly all plastic lens materials will absorb this dye, except for polycarbonate and Trivex. (Even in those cases, the lens coating will absorb some dye.)

The third way of producing a fixed lens color is with a **laminated** lens. This is where the lens has a colored layer affixed to one surface, and this is commonly found with modern polarized sun lenses.

Protecting the Eye from UV Exposure

The optical components of the eye, like any delicate structure, are subject to damage by prolonged exposure to ultraviolet radiation. One has only to observe the yellowing of an old car's headlight lens to see this effect. UV exposure has been linked to corneal conditions, cataract formation, and even retinal damage. Therefore, it makes sense to protect the eye from as much of this radiation as possible.

When in prolonged periods of outdoor activity, a good pair of sunglasses with at least a 95% UV-blocking lens is always recommended. Ordinary dress eyewear is almost always insufficient, even with photochromatic lenses, because everyday eyewear will often allow enough ambient light from above and to the side to cause damage. A fully darkened Transitions lens will block around 95%, and most polycarbonate and high-index lenses block 100% of UV light by nature. (Even CR-39 can be treated to block nearly that much.) But enough light always gets around such lenses to cause damage anyway, especially at places like the beach, where the sand scatters the UV light in all directions.

Antireflective Coating

Antireflective (AR) coatings (often called nonglare) have been around for years, in professional applications such as camera lenses and telescope optics, for the simple reason that they improve the clarity and effectiveness of the lens. Any eyeglass lens will reflect away some amount of the light striking it, anywhere from 8% and up to 15% or more on the higher index materials. An AR coating will reduce this reflectivity down to as low as 0.5%, meaning that more of the light gets through to the eye.

The primary factor holding back patient acceptance of AR coatings as a useful feature has always been its own delicacy. They can be hard to clean and to keep clean, and they are often easily damaged if overcleaned. Thus, the most important advance in AR coatings was to make them user-friendly. More modern coatings are being produced with multiple additional layers of protection, such as a **hydrophobic** top coat (which repels water) and **oleophobic** top coats (which repel oils from the skin, keeping the lens from smudging in the first place). Neglecting these features is often a recipe for a patient complaint, and he may even wind up back in the office to ask that you remove the coating.

Mirror Coatings

Mirror coatings have been around for a long time and are often used for various cosmetic reasons. But in fact, there is a definite science behind these coatings.

The observed color of a mirror coating represents the wavelengths of light that do not penetrate it. This means that a reddish-tinted mirrored lens is keeping reds and infrareds out of the patient's eyes. Because the eye has no way of cooling itself, attenuating the infrared can help the eyes keep from feeling gritty and tired. Likewise, a blue mirror is keeping blues and high-energy violet light out of the eye, which not only minimizes ocular damage from these rays, but enhances contrast, because blue light is the most easily scattered color. A gold mirror will reduce the overall intensity of the visual image, because the eye normally perceives yellow as the brightest color. Silver being neutral, a mirror of that hue will merely add to the overall light-blocking characteristics of the lens.

Frame Considerations for Younger Patients

Young patients' needs change dramatically as they grow. For example, with extremely young wearers, one of the primary concerns is how to keep the frame on the child's face. This can be accomplished by the use of frames that can be held in place by elastic straps or by using cable temples to grip the ears. Soft frame materials are a good choice for this age bracket, as are frames with a saddle fit and no nose pads to injure them if something strikes them in the face. Once a child is old enough to understand that he must keep the glasses on, the more common skull-fit temples may be sufficient.

Toddlers are still very active little people and can still be injured by nose pads if they happen to fall down. This makes a plastic frame the safer choice, in many cases.

As children age, they become extremely style conscious and will often prefer frame styles and designs that they see their friends or their heroes wear. This factor becomes very obvious as they become teenagers, and it may be wise for the parents to let the child choose what she wants, simply to ensure that the eyewear will be worn.

Influence of Prescription Values on Choice of Frame Shape

The experienced optician can look at a patient's prescription and immediately know what the shape of the lens will be. This can help her steer the patient away from frame shapes that would naturally accentuate thickness at prominent points.

As an example, a patient with strong cylinder power at axes close to the horizontal will have lenses that quickly get thick at the top and bottom. Therefore, a very tall lens shape makes a poor choice, whereas a skinnier shape will produce thinner edges. Likewise, the same kind of Rx with axes at 45 and 135 will produce thickening at the upper temporal corners, which will be emphasized by prominent corners in the frame shape, or conversely minimized by a rounder shape.

Frame Considerations When Fitting Progressive-Addition Multifocals

Modern progressive multifocals come in a large variety of add-corridor lengths, so it is important to choose a frame with enough depth to handle the full length of the corridor that you will be using, without crowding the patient's distance vision too much.

Also, a frame that sits too close to the cheek at the bottom can render the strongest parts of the corridor useless, because the patient will never look far enough down to see it. This is especially true of saddle-fit plastic frames, unless proper attention is paid to the way it sits on the patient's bridge.

Semirimless frames can also be a problem with progressive lenses, simply because the variable shape of the lens surface creates a thinner lens at the bottom than at the top, precisely where edge thickness can be a problem. Polycarbonate lens material can help avoid the chipping problem, but even so, you might wind up having to thicken the entire lens just to accommodate a bottom edge that is thick enough to hold a groove.

Factors That Guide Frame Selection for Very High Prescriptions

The first consideration in frame selection for high prescriptions is the overall size of the lens. In general, a smaller shape is preferable to a larger shape because a smaller shape will produce thinner edge profiles or center thickness.

Secondly, one must consider how the **frame PD** compares to the patient's PD. Frame PD is defined as the distance between the geometric centers of the lenses, usually measured from the nasal edge of one lens to the temporal edge of the other. The more decentration that will be required when edging lenses at the patient's PD, the greater the unwanted edge or center thickness will be.

Finally, one must consider frame construction. Whereas a plastic frame will hide some of the lens thickness, a rimless or semirimless style will show it off and may even add thickness (such as a higher plus lens in a semirimless frame, which requires a minimum edge thickness for the groove). Even if the patient is accepting of the appearance, a very thick lens in a rimless frame may end up excessively front heavy, whereas a plastic or metal full-rim frame may distribute the weight more evenly.

Critical Factors in Choosing Best-Fitting Frames

The most critical three factors in achieving frame comfort are bridge fit, frame width, and temple length.

A good bridge fit can be accomplished with a plastic frame if attention is paid to the shape and strength of the patient's nose. Most plastics are called saddle-fit bridges for a good reason — the frame should match the curve of the patient's nose and mate with it, like a saddle on a horse. Less commonly, a plastic frame will have a keyhole bridge, where only the sides are meant to come into contact with the nose, but these should also seat solidly. If the patient's does not have a strong enough nose shape, a metal frame with adjustable pads might provide the better bridge fit.

Frame width is measured from the tip of one end piece to the other. A frame with adequate width will allow the temples to go straight back, grazing the head just in front of the ears.

Temple length should be enough to provide adequate holding power behind the ear. A temple should be long enough to wrap down behind the ear (a skull fit) or partway around the back of the head (an occipital fit).

Influence of Lens Material on Frame Construction and Vice Versa

Lens material and frame construction should go hand in hand. Sometimes, one will dictate the other.

If a patient wants to choose a rimless or semirimless frame style, for example, he should always be steered toward more durable lens materials than plastic. A semirimless frame usually requires a grooved-edge lens, which holds a nylon filament tightly around it. Especially at the thinnest lens edge, this groove can chip and break out with a plastic lens. The other kind of semirimless mounting, with a notched frame body and hooked lens shape, is even more unforgiving of plastic. Polycarbonate and Trivex are always more acceptable choices, in both cases.

With drill-mounted rimless eyewear, we are asking the lens to provide some of the structural support that the frame will not, and tougher lens materials become an absolute must. Again, polycarbonate and Trivex are good choices, although high-index lenses also bear up well in these frames.

Patient-Driven Considerations When Choosing a Base Curve as Part of the Overall Lens Design

Besides pure optics, there are a few other considerations at play when choosing the appropriate base curve for a lens. Steeper base curves tend to produce a greater magnification effect, making them cosmetically unappealing and visually disorienting for the patient, and so a flatter-than-ideal lens is often the goal. And with many of today's sportier wrapped sunglass frames, a much steeper than normal base curve is required, regardless of the prescription. Thus, the choice of base curvature becomes a complex balance of concerns, including perfect-world optics, patient needs, frame requirements, and final cosmetics.

Fitting Height of Multifocal Lens

The fitting height of a multifocal lens refers to the physical positioning of the reading area within the lens.

In order to produce maximum usability for the patient, the near-vision portion of the lens must be located in a natural-feeling position, so that in situations where his eyes might normally go to something nearby (such as a book or a phone), the necessary power will be in the right place. In general, segmented bifocals and trifocals are positioned low in the lens, whereas progressive multifocals are positioned higher in the lens.

The positioning within the frame is determined with the patient in front of the dispenser and a reference point being marked on the lens. Each lens type has a suggested typical reference point: bifocals at the lower lid, trifocals at the bottom of the pupil, progressives at the pupillary center. But none of these guidelines is absolute, and the optician is responsible for using his judgment, based on the patient's intended use of the eyewear as well as his wearing history.

OC Height

In multifocal height measurement, the position of the optical center (OC) is generally left at a standard measurement above the segment line. (With progressive lenses, the fitting height and OC height are the same.) When fitting a single bifocal or trifocal lens, the OC height of the opposite lens should be measured and matched.

In single-vision lenses, the OC height should be taken and used if it varies significantly from the geometric center of the lens. In this case, the OC height is defined as either a distance above the geometric center or above the bottom of the frame. The OC height can be especially important when fitting lenses with a higher refractive index, in order to provide the best optics at the patient's eye level.

Image Jump

When the patient is looking through the optical center of the lens, there is no extra prism displacement beyond any in the prescription. Once she looks away from the center, this changes, but in a gradual way that she does not perceive.

A segmented multifocal of any kind interrupts this peaceful arrangement. Once the patient's view touches the edge of the segment, there will be a sudden increase in induced prism, based on the power of the segment itself. The resulting sudden shift is called image jump.

The amount of image jump in a multifocal lens will depend on the design of the add segment. Every segment has its own optical center, and the distance of that center from the edge of the segment can be inserted into the Prentice formula, using the power of the segment to calculate the prism at its edge. Round segments are the worst because the eye must travel the farthest to reach the segment's OC. Flat-top segments are a little better because the upper part of the add lens has been cut away.

Relationship Between Refractive Index and Final Lens Appearance

In general, a minus lens with a higher Rx will produce thick edges, whereas a strong plus lens will produce a thick center. This can be mitigated greatly by the use of a lens with a higher refractive index.

A polycarbonate lens, with an index of 1.58, will reduce the edge thickness of a minus lens by roughly one-third. Pushing the index up above 1.70 will reduce the thickness by nearly 50%. Because the cost goes up with the refractive index whereas optical clarity goes down, aesthetics must always be weighed against these other factors; the best trade-off is the one that meets all of these needs in the middle.

Usefulness of Various Lens Tints

A dark lens tint is typically used to create a sunglass effect. Dark browns, grays, and greens are the most common colors for this purpose. Either way, the primary effect is to increase the patient's comfort in bright sunlight. But the three differ somewhat in their function. The gray lens is neutral, darkening everything evenly across the spectrum, but its effect weakens a bit toward the violet end of the spectrum. The brown lens counters this by negating the violet end, increasing contrast in the process but allowing some infrareds to pass. The green lens is almost in the middle of the visible spectrum, and it covers undesirable wavelengths at both ends, although many patients find the resulting coloring objectionable.

Lighter tints have various other uses. Light browns and ambers are good at enhancing contrast, because they block out light-scattering blue wavelengths. Yellow is excellent for nighttime driving, both for its contrast-enhancing ability and the way it does not darken the rest of the spectrum. Pink tints were widely used in the early days of computers, to soften the green characters on a black screen, but this is no longer the concern it once was, except in certain industrial applications.

Benefits of Antireflective Coating

From the patient's perspective, only a maximum of about 92% of the light striking his lenses actually reaches his eyes. The rest is either scattered between the front and back surfaces of the lens or bounced away entirely. This not only reduces the available light to see with, it can also produce annoying and distracting reflections, especially when driving into headlights on a rainy night. The antireflective coating dramatically reduces these problems by allowing nearly all of the ambient light to pass through the lens. More light is made available to the eyes, and distracting reflections are eliminated.

Visible Result and Benefits of Looking Through a Polarized Lens

A lens that is merely dark tinted will pass whatever light is available to it, reduced by whatever percentage of light it normally blocks. But not all light is beneficial. The **polarized lens** eliminates light reflected horizontally from shiny surfaces, such as car windows, wet roads, and bodies of water. This often results in a more accurate picture of what is in front of the patient, and it can make daytime driving a much safer experience. It can also make beachgoing much more comfortable. Fishermen often love this lens, because it allows them to see directly into the water, rather than being blinded by the reflection of the sky. The polarization is accomplished by a laminated layer on the front or back surface of the lens.

Questions to Help Patient Discuss His Own Needs

An optician might ask the patient, what do you do for a living, Mr. Jones? This invites the patient to tell you how he spends his typical day. Asking, do you have any hobbies, Mrs. Smith? gives her an opportunity to open up about what she likes to do in her free time. The question, where is your ideal vacation? might open up a conversation about new activities that the patient would like to be prepared for. Do you have any time of the day when your eyes always get feeling tired? is a good way to find the weaknesses in the patient's existing visual strategy.

Helping Patients Understand Daily Demands on Vision

The eyes have a lot of work to do in the course of a day, and it is the optician's job to discover when the patient is placing the heaviest demand on them. A computer operator, for example, spends the majority of his or her day staring at a screen 30 inches away. An electrician might spend a good share of the day peering into circuit breaker panels and reading fine print. A construction foreman might spend most of his day squinting out in the blazing sun. Each of these constitutes a high-demand activity for the eyes, but the patient may not even realize it until you point it out to him, after getting him to talk about his daily activity. Zero in on those high-demand areas, and you will have pinpointed how to best help the patient.

Suggesting Lens Types and Options to Enhance Patient's Lifestyle

A patient who does a lot of daytime driving would benefit from a pair of polarized sunglasses. Mr. Jones, how would you like to cut down the glare of the sun and clarify your vision through the windshield? A patient who spends most of his day in front of a computer would benefit from a pair of intermediate-vision glasses. Mrs. Smith, how would you like for your eyes not to be so tired at the end of the workday? A patient who has trouble with nighttime driving would benefit from an antireflective coating. Bob, how would you like to make your nighttime vision clearer and easier on your eyes?

Lens Availability Limitations

Not every lens is available with every option imaginable. Often, the less-popular lens styles will have many gaps, in which a desired option is simply not offered. This frequently occurs with some of the older segmented multifocals, but even in progressive lenses, you will often find that one lens will offer certain combinations of options and another will not. A good example is high-index lenses with photochromatics. One progressive lens might be available all the way up to 1.74 index with a Transitions option, whereas another might only offer Transitions up to 1.60 index.

A good way to work around such limitations is to always have a backup plan. If a patient is looking for the thinnest lens available but also wants a photochromatic lens, offer his first progressive lens choice in the highest index to include both, as well as an alternative lens that may be more expensive but offer a photochromatic 1.74 index. That way, the patient makes the final call.

Discouraging Patients from Buying Particular Lens Option

Not all lens options are the best for all patients, and anytime a patient is asking for something that will not benefit him, it is smart to explain why, and talk the patient out of it if possible.

A good example is the patient who states he is looking for a Transitions lens so that he will have sunglasses when he is driving. It is a good optician's duty to point out to this patient that the lens he plans to spend so much money on will not change color very much behind the windshield. He would be better served by a dedicated pair of polarized sunglasses.

Another case would be a patient who wants a pair of polarized sunwear but intends to use them primarily to read liquid crystal display screens, such as a deepwater fisherman who uses a depth-finding app on his laptop. He will curse the optician who sold him that pair, when it causes his laptop's screen to blank out. His optimal pair of sunglasses would be a dark charcoal-brown tint with a blue mirror coating.

Bench Aligning a Frame

A frame can be said to be in **bench alignment** or **four-point alignment** when it will sit upside-down on a flat surface with all four points in contact with the surface, and the temples pointing straight back from the frame corners.

The optician should start at the bridge, making sure it is straight and that the lenses are in **coplanar alignment** (not twisted in an X to each other). This should leave the frame front in a slight inward face-form curvature, or straight across, but never bent backwards. The end pieces and hinges should then be positioned to give the frame front about an 8- to 10-degree **pantoscopic tilt**, inward from the vertical at the lens bottom.

The end pieces should be further adjusted to bring the temples parallel with each other, pointing straight back. Finally, the hinges and temples should be adjusted to present an identical appearance and to make contact with the table equally to each other.

Final Verification of a Pair of Single-Vision Eyewear

Final verification of all eyewear is done at a lensometer. It is recommended to always begin not with the right lens, but the lens of stronger power.

With that lens in position, use the power and axis drums to dial in the expected power and axis. Center the lens image within the reticle, and move the frame table up to meet the frame. Gently clamp the lens in place. Observe the centered image, noting any deviations from powers or axis. (Refer to the ANSI Z80.1 standards for acceptable deviation.) Dot the lens with the spotting pins.

Without moving the frame table, unclamp the eyewear and move to the opposite lens, centering that image in the reticle. Note any vertical deviation. Dial in the expected powers and axis, noting any deviations, and dot the second lens. Remove the eyewear from the lensometer, measure the distances of the dots from the center of the bridge, and compare these to the patient's monocular PDs. (Refer to the ANSI Z80.1 standards for acceptable deviations.)

Final Verification of a Pair of Segmented Multifocal Eyewear

Final verification of all eyewear is done at a lensometer, beginning with the lens of stronger power.

Use the power and axis drums to dial in the expected power and axis of the first lens. Center the image within the reticle, and move the frame table up to meet the frame. Gently clamp the lens in place. Observe the centered image, noting any deviations from powers or axis. Dot the lens with the spotting pins. Now unclamp the lens, move the power drum to increase it to the anticipated sphere + add power, and raise the lens to verify the resulting power at the segment. The most accurate reading will be from the back of the lens.

Without moving the frame table, move to the opposite lens, repeating the above procedure. Note any vertical deviation in the distance centration. Remove the eyewear from the lensometer, measure the separation of the dots from each other, and compare this to the patient's binocular PD. Note the relationship of distance centers to segment lines, which should match. Note the distance between segments, which should correspond to the patient's near PD. Note the height of the segments from the bottom of the frame. (Refer to the ANSI Z80.1 standards for all acceptable deviations.)

Final Verification of Eyewear with a Pair of Progressive-Addition Lenses

Beginning with the stronger lens, use the power and axis drums to dial in the expected power and axis. Locate the center spotting pin at the manufacturer's reference point, and gently clamp the lens in place. The image will appear off-power, but note its position. Repeat this with the opposite lens, and note any deviation from matched or **yoked** displacement.

Return to the first lens, centering the lensometer within the manufacturer's distance verification circle above the fitting cross, raising the frame table and gently clamping the eyewear in place. Observe the off-centered image, noting any deviations from powers or axis. Now unclamp the lens, move the power drum to increase it to the anticipated sphere + add power, and raise the lens to the lower verification circle to verify the resulting power at the bottom of the corridor.

Move to the opposite lens, repeating the above procedure. Then remove the eyewear from the lensometer, measure the distance of the major reference points (MRPs) from the center of the bridge, and compare this to the patient's monocular PDs. Note the heights of the fitting crosses from the bottom of the frame. (Refer to the ANSI Z80.1 standards for all acceptable deviations.)

Verifying the Prescribed Prism in a Finished Pair of Single-Vision Glasses

When the prescription is calling for ground-in prism, the object is to determine the amount of dioptric deviation from normal centration. This will be measured at the lensometer by the position of the mires within the reticle.

For a single-vision lens, one must first mark the desired PD onto the lens, and that becomes the point of reference. In a single-vision prescription with a specified prism value in the right lens of three diopters base-in, for example, we would begin with the left eye, centering the mires vertically and horizontally at the point called for by the PD. Then (without moving the frame table), move the right lens into position so that the PD mark is centered with the spotting pin. Rotate the reticle so that the line is horizontal. The mires should converge along the line where it intersects the three-diopter circle, offset toward the patient's nose. Any deviation of more than one-third diopter from this is unacceptable.

Verifying Prescribed Prism in a Finished Pair of Segmented-Multifocal Glasses

When the prescription is calling for ground-in prism, the object is to determine the amount of dioptric deviation from normal **centration**. This will be measured at the **lensometer** by the position of the **mires** within the **reticle**. But the point of reference on the lens is the key, and it must be established first.

For a lined multifocal, the point of reference will be determined both by the specified distance of the optical center above the reading segment (typically 3–5 mm) and by the inset of the segment to accommodate near convergence (typically 1–2 mm). Once the "normal" location of the OC is established, the prism would be measured using that point of reference. In a prescription with a specified prism value in the right lens of three diopters base-in, for example, we would move the right lens into position so that the established reference point is centered with the spotting pin. Rotate the reticle so that the line is horizontal. The mires should converge along the line where it intersects the three-diopter circle, offset toward the patient's nose. Any deviation of more than one-third diopter from this is unacceptable.

Verifying Prescribed Prism in a Finished Pair of Progressive Multifocal Glasses

When the prescription is calling for ground-in prism, the object is to determine the amount of dioptric deviation from normal centration. This will be measured at the lensometer by the position of the mires within the reticle.

On a marked lens such as a progressive, the central dot or **manufacturer's reference point** (MRP) is used, by locating the central spotting pin at that point. (The power of the lens at that MRP is irrelevant; we are only noting its location.) For both lenses, the mires would then normally appear off center by the same amount, commonly downward from center by 0.5 or so. If the left-eye Rx calls for prism of 2 diopters base-down, begin with the right lens, centering it on the MRP, and noting the mires' position within the reticle. (We'll assume 0.5 down, for this example.) Then, without moving the frame table, center the left lens at the MRP. Rotate the reticle so that the 180-degree line is vertical. The mires should converge on it, halfway between the 2- and 3-diopter circles below center (0.5 + 2 = 2.5). Any deviation of more than 1/3 diopter from this is unacceptable.

Solutions Employed by Different Lensometer Styles for Coping with Extreme Prismatic Image Displacement

The reticle in the average lensometer is designed to locate an image prismed out to about 5 diopters in any direction. Beyond that amount of prism, the image may fall outside the reticle or even beyond the field of view entirely.

The solution for this on older instruments was the addition of **auxiliary prism rings** to the back of the eyepiece. These came in sets of 3.00, 6.00, and 9.00 D, and the optician would use whichever one brought the image closest to center, calculating any remaining displacement against the value of the ring. Rotating the ring would change the direction of the prism displacement.

On many newer models, there will be a **prism compensator** built into the eyepiece. Rotating the knob will decenter the image further and further, whereas moving it around the axis of the eyepiece will reposition the direction of the prism. This can be used in two ways: either the expected prism and direction can be set beforehand and the lens can then be checked for visible centration in the reticle; or the lens can be positioned at the desired physical point, the compensator adjusted until the image is centered, and the values read on the compensator's scale.

Importance of Matching All Elements of Patient's Order to the Finished Product

There are so many considerations having to do purely with the optics of the eyewear, it is easy to overlook other issues just as critical. For instance, if you have ordered eyewear for a husband and wife, and the optics are pristine but his Rx has been mounted into her frame, the entire process fails. The patient will never see and may not notice a three-degree axis error, but they are certain to notice a frame that is pink instead of gunmetal.

Look at the frame: Does it match what the patient selected, for model and color? If the lens was ordered as photochromatic, did it arrive that way? Are the bifocal segments lined up straight? Was the antireflective coating applied? Did the lab give you the correct lens style? Unlike the optical tolerances, these are all issues that the patient will spot in a flash, and they are no less important to the end product.

Instrumentation

Lens Clock

The **lens clock**, sometimes called the **spherometer** or the **Geneva Lens Measure**, is a small tool with a dial gauge that is used to measure the curvature(s) of a lens. There will be three pins along one edge; the outer two are fixed, and the inner one is movable. Holding the clock perpendicular to the lens, the pins are pressed against the center of the lens surface. The black numbers on the dial are for plus curvature readings, whereas the red numbers are for minus readings.

The lens clock is most often used to determine the base curvature of an existing lens, for purposes of matching it on the new eyewear. This is important if the patient has gotten used to a particular curvature or when ordering lenses for a wrapped sunglass frame. It can also be used to read the **surface power** of a lens, by taking the front and back curves and combining them algebraically.

The lens clock's highly accurate big brother, the **sagitta gauge**, is used to measure the precise base curvature of a lens blank in order to calculate the necessary back curvatures for surfacing, taking the refractive index into account.

Determining Single-Vision Lens Powers on a Lensometer

The lens is placed in front of the main lensometer element, and then it is adjusted to produce an image centered in the reticle, as viewed through the eyepiece. Begin by rotating the power drum all the way to the plus end (usually the numbers in black), and then slowly rotate backward until an image comes into focus. Note the power that the indicator is pointing to. This is the sphere power of the lens.

If the lens is other than spherical, the image will not fully resolve until the axis drum is turned. Rotate this drum until the skinny lines are all aligned in sharp focus. (Microadjust the power drum if necessary.) Then rotate the power drum further toward the minus end until the thick lines come into focus. Note the difference between the two powers on the drum, and this becomes the cylinder power of the lens.

If a plus-cylinder Rx is desired, reverse the operation, first rotating the power drum all the way minus, then backward to find the sphere power, and finally rotating it further plus to find the cylinder power.

Methods Used in Reading Multifocal Powers on a Lensometer

With a multifocal lens, the distance prescription must first be determined, following the procedure for a single-vision lens. Note the sphere power of the lens. Then move the lens so as to place the reading area in front of the main lensometer element. Rotate the power drum toward the plus side until the image comes back into focus. Note the difference between this power and the sphere power. This becomes the add power of the lens.

When measuring add powers on a segmented multifocal, it is generally recommended to reverse the lens, reading it from the back as opposed to from the front. This is because the increased distance of the segment from the lensometer optics can have a small but measurable **vertex effect**, causing the add power to read too high. The higher the lens powers, the greater the effect.

When measuring add powers (or any powers) on a progressive lens, always read the lens within the manufacturer's verification circles, for greatest accuracy.

Verifying PD and Unwanted Prism at the Lensometer

When placing the finished eyewear in the lensometer, the image is generally centered within the reticle. The spotting pins are used to mark this centered position on the lens (the optical center), and the distance from this mark to the center of the bridge of the frame (for monocular measurements) or to the opposite lens' optical center (for binocular measurements) is measured and compared to the patient's pupillary distance. Ideally, this will match within 2 mm. If it does not, there are two methods for determining whether the glasses are acceptable:

Use a marker to indicate the point on the lens where the expected PD would fall, center the lens spotting pin at this point, and observe the amount of unwanted prism indicated within the reticle. More than one-third diopter is unacceptable.

Note the difference between the expected PD and the actual PD. Apply the Prentice formula to determine the amount of unwanted prism. For example, if the PD is off by 4 mm (0.4 cm) and the lens power is −3.00, the formula would read $0.4 \times 3.00 = 1.2$ diopters of prism, and the glasses are out of tolerance.

Use of Pupillometer to Measure a Patient's PD

With the patient sitting at eye level to the optician, the pupillometer is gently pressed against the patient's bridge, making sure the eyes are level with the pupillometer lenses. Have the patient look directly at the lighted target. The optician then observes the reflected spot of light on the patient's cornea and lines up the crosshair with the spot. The pupillary distance is then read on the top of the instrument, either on an analog scale or in a digital readout.

Measurements Obtained Using the Pupillometer

Most modern pupillometers will give a total of three readings. The reading for each individual eye is called the **monocular PD**, and it indicates the distance from the pupil center to the bridge of the nose. The combined reading for both eyes is called the **binocular PD**, and it is the same measurement that would be produced by measuring from eye to eye with a ruler.

There are many uses for both types of PD measurement, and the optician will need to make the call as to which is more appropriate.

Measuring a Near PD Using a Pupillometer

The modern pupillometer includes a way to simulate different viewing distances, producing a measurement appropriate to the application.

The default setting is always infinity, or a viewing distance at which the visual axes are nearly parallel. But when looking at a phone or reading a magazine, the eyes move closer together. The patient's natural near convergence can be simulated with the pupillometer, by changing the setting to 35–40 cm, a typical near range. The PD measurement obtained with this setting will always be about 3–4 mm less than the distance PD obtained at the infinity setting.

Measuring a Vertex Distance

The patient's fitted **vertex** is the distance from the cornea to the back of the lens. This can be roughly estimated using a PD ruler, by holding it up to the patient's temple while he is wearing the frame, lining up the zero point with the front of the eye, and measuring to the plane of the demo lens.

A more accurate measurement may be taken with the **distometer**. This device is used with the frame on but the patient's eye closed. Inserted between the frame and the eye, it is gently opened up until it touches the back of the lens and the patient's closed eyelid. The exact vertex measurement is then read on a scale.

Frame Warmer

The frame warmer is used to assist in lens insertions into plastic frames and to soften and reform portions of the frame during final adjustment.

Plastic frames require that the lens be pushed into the frame, which forces the frame to stretch a bit. Depending on the thickness of the frame material, this can be somewhat difficult, and it is made much easier by softening the frame with a little heat. In extreme cases (such as sport goggles), the frame must be heated to very high temperatures. In other cases in which the frame material is lighter gauge, care must be taken not to overheat the frame and cause shrinkage or deformity.

Plastic frames are also adjusted in the same manner — by heating and reforming the area that needs it. Metal frames are generally only heated at the temple tips, which usually have a plastic covering.

The two types of frame warmers are the pan type and hot-air warmers. The pan type will be filled with glass beads or salt heated to a high temperature, and the frame must be swirled through the heated grains. The hot-air warmer blows a focused stream of heated air that can be applied to the frame where necessary.

Frame Material with Which Frame Warmer Should Be Used with Utmost Caution

There are two types of plastic frame material that can easily be destroyed by careless heating. Fortunately, they are seldom used anymore. Unfortunately, this makes a mistake easier to happen when they do appear.

Very thin plastic frames, manufactured under names like SPX and Grilamid, can be ruined by overheating. Often, the manufacturers would recommend cold insertion of the lenses. But even these frames need occasional adjustments. Use extreme caution because just a little too much heat will cause them to deform or shrink beyond usability.

Optyl frames can be heated safely, but although they may stretch, they will never shrink back to their original size. What's more, when they change from semiliquid back to solid, they undergo a structural change at the molecular level that momentarily makes them brittle. Attempting to flex them during cooling will result in the material snapping like a strand of uncooked spaghetti — a very unfortunate situation for any optician.

Lens Coating That Can Be Damaged by the Frame Warmer

Besides abrasion, antireflective coatings have one major enemy: high heat. It will cause the coating to **craze**, creating the appearance of a fine spiderweb of small cracks. These may be hard to see inside the office, but the patient will notice them immediately when he or she walks out into the sunlight.

For this reason, anytime you are heating a plastic frame to adjust it anywhere near the eyewire, it is highly recommended to remove an antireflective-coated lens, and reinsert it afterward. Always be sure, of course, to verify the orientation of the lens after doing so.

Common Tools for Adjusting Metal Frames

Probably the most commonly used tool on the optician's bench is a good pair of **nose pad pliers**. These pliers have one flat jaw and one with a small box shape to support the end of the nose pad arm, allowing for easy adjusting without putting undue stress on the pads themselves.

Another indispensable tool is the **half-round pliers**. These pliers will have one round jaw and one flat jaw, and they are usually padded with nylon on the flat side. Their function is in gripping and adjusting the frame at tight spots such as the corners in front of the hinges, without leaving a mark.

One of the oldest yet handiest tools is the **Numont pliers**. This tool comes with a small channel cut across the tips of both jaws, and it is used for steadying one part of the frame while bending another very close to it. They are also useful for holding a screw by the head to hold it steady for insertion.

The **angling pliers** are for adjusting pantoscopic tilt. Often used in tandem with the Numont pliers, they will firmly grip the end piece or hinge to angle it downward or upward, increasing or decreasing the tilt of the frame front.

Common Tools for Adjusting Plastic Frames

Plastic frames are much softer than metal frames, particularly when heated, and so the tools needed to adjust them need to protect against permanent denting and marring.

Probably the most common tool used on plastic frames is the **double-padded pliers**. These have two flat jaws with nylon covering on both sides. They are a good multipurpose tool for angling and forming at the temples and corners.

A variation on the half-round pliers, the nylon-jawed **Zyl-gripping pliers** are padded on one side and metal on the other, but both sides are flat. This tool is used to grip and safely adjust a plastic frame at the hinge, with the metal side in contact with the back of the hinge body and the wide nylon-padded side protecting the outside of the end piece or temple.

Seldom seen anymore, **bridge-stretching pliers** are used for exactly what the name describes, when a plastic frame is slightly too narrow for the patient's nose. It has two sets of large, rounded pins to grip at both ends of the bridge, and it will safely stretch a heated plastic bridge a few millimeters.

Hand Tools Used in Lab Setting

Some tools are best left on the bench, to be used during fabrication and assembly rather than for making adjustments in front of the patient, who may find them unnerving.

A good example of these is the **end-cutting** or **Chappel pliers**. This versatile tool is commonly used to cut off unnecessarily long screws, when replacing hinge screws, or when assembling nut-and-bolt rimless eyewear. The sound they make will often give the patient the impression that something is being broken.

Compression pliers (which come in several variations) are used to assemble compression-mounted rimless eyewear. Ideally, they will make no sound, but this is still not an operation that the average patient wishes to see.

Axis pliers are for gripping the lens and rotating it slightly, to correct an axis error. This is a risky procedure that can easily scratch a lens, and it is something that should be done well before the patient arrives.

Less common are **eyewire-shaping pliers**, which have jaws that are convex on one side and concave on the other, with nylon padding on both sides. It can be used to gently form a distorted metal eyewire back into shape without leaving a crease or marring the surface but this all happens prior to mounting the lens.

Changing Pantoscopic Tilt on Plastic Frames

On any frame, there are two places of adjustment where the pantoscopic tilt may be changed: at the end pieces of the frame front or at the hinges.

With a plastic frame, the easiest place to adjust is at the hinge, provided you can do so without creating an unappealing gap. The front half of the hinge should be stabilized using the nylon-jaw Zyl-gripping pliers, with the metal jaw firmly against the front of the hinge. Using either a pair of double-nylon-jaw adjusting pliers or the angling pliers, grip the temple behind the hinge. Bend downward to increase the pantoscopic tilt or upward to reduce it.

It is more difficult to do so, but if there is sufficient flexibility at the end pieces, that is the more elegant place to make this adjustment. Doing so avoids the risk of damaging or loosening the hinge, and it will never cause a hinge gap. Heat the end pieces to soften them, and then use nylon adjusting pliers or a tabletop to form them in the proper direction. You may need to rewiden the temples afterward, because this adjustment often brings them inward.

Changing Pantoscopic Tilt on Metal Frames

On any frame, there are two places of adjustment where the pantoscopic tilt may be changed: at the end pieces of the frame front or at the hinges. Metal frames simultaneously offer more and less flexibility than plastic frames — more, in that it is often easier to bend them where you want to go and make them stay, and less, in that the material itself is frequently less malleable than heated plastic.

The easiest place to adjust is at the hinge, provided you can do so without creating an unappealing gap. The front half of the hinge should be stabilized with nylon-padded half-round pliers, with the nylon jaw on the outside of the frame to avoid marring it. The angling pliers can then be used to turn the temple side of the hinge downward to increase the pantoscopic tilt, or upward to decrease it.

If there is sufficient end piece to do so, adjusting the end piece rather than the hinge provides the most stable positioning of all. Use the Numont pliers to firmly stabilize the part of the end piece facing forward, and then use the angling pliers to grip the part leading toward the temples, bending it downward or upward as needed.

Lens Caliper

The **lens caliper**, sometimes simply called the lens thickness gauge, is a tool for checking lens thickness. Most are simple devices — two nylon-tipped jaws that read on a scale when opened. More complicated versions may have a dial gauge that gives a more precise reading.

Lenses must be dispensed within minimum center thickness standards, and these can be verified using the lens caliper. This tool is also used when heat-tempering a glass lens, by measuring the thinnest and thickest points and averaging them, to calculate an optimum heating time.

Polariscope

The **polariscope** is used to detect stresses within the structure of a lens. This is important after heat-tempering glass lenses, to ensure that the proper stress pattern has been created to avoid shattering. It is also used to prevent overtightening of a lens in an eyewire, by showing a stress pattern where there should be none.

A polariscope is nothing more than two polarizing filters at 90 degrees to each other. Portable versions flip open, and the filters are placed either side of the lens, whereas tabletop versions will have a light mounted underneath the two filters.

First Procedure When Beginning Work at a Lensometer

The most often overlooked operation to perform at the lensometer is that of first zeroing the eyepiece. To accommodate small variations in the vision from one optician to another, the eyepiece has a small amount of ± adjustment available. This is best done prior to looking at the first lens.

First, the power drum is rotated away from zero to defocus the image of the mires, leaving only the reticle visible. Next, the eyepiece is rotated slowly back and forth until the reticle is at its sharpest focus. The lensometer should now be ready for the optician to use, obtaining the most accurate results.

Correcting for Small Zeroing Errors at the Power Drum

Occasionally, you will find that a lensometer is not coming into plano focus with the power drum reading exactly at zero. This can throw off every power reading the optician makes, by as much as 0.25. Fortunately, this problem can often be corrected at the drum itself, or rather at the pointer next to the drum.

With the lensometer in plano focus, use a screwdriver or hex wrench to loosen the screws holding the pointer in place. Using care not to move the power drum, position the pointer so that it aims precisely at 0. Carefully retighten the screws, with the pointer in its new position. The lensometer should now read accurately.

Correcting a Power Error That Increases with the Strength of the Prescription

If the lensometer consistently displays a progressive power error in high prescriptions — that is, if the higher the Rx, the more pronounced the error — then it is in need of a vertex adjustment. This is done at the **lens stop**, the aperture directly in front of the primary optics.

The vertex effect dictates that a minus lens that is further from the eye (or in this case, the optics) produces a weaker effective power, whereas a plus lens will produce a greater effective power. Therefore, moving the lens stop closer to the primary optics will strengthen a high-minus power and weaken a high-plus power. Using a small hex wrench (typically), loosen the set screw holding the lens stop in place. Rotate it clockwise to increase a high-minus overpower reading or decrease a high-plus underpower reading. Rotate it counterclockwise for the opposite problem. Move it only one rotation at a time, using a set of calibrated test lenses to verify when the power is reading correctly. Double-check the powers on the opposite end, and then retighten the set screw when both are reading as accurately as possible.

Periodic Care Given to Instrument Optics

There are many optical elements in a lensometer, but most are well hidden and out of harm's way. The major exception to this is the eyepiece. If the eyepiece gets dirty and smudged, nothing else will look right. Therefore, it makes sense to keep the eyepiece clean.

Visually inspect the eyepiece daily, and look for signs of smudges or dust. The eyepiece has an antireflective (AR) coating on it, which should be handled with just as much care as a patient's AR-coated lenses. Gently clean the eyepiece with a soft cloth, using a dab of alcohol as necessary to eliminate any oils. Dry it immediately after, using another area of the cloth.

The same thing applies to pupillometer lenses, which are prone to picking up oils from patients' faces or from general handling. These also will have an AR coating, and they should be cleaned just as gently.

If a protective cover is available for either of these devices, keeping it on when they are not in use will greatly reduce the buildup of dust on the optics, which will reduce the need to clean them.

Sanitizing Tools and Equipment

Any piece of equipment in any doctor's office that comes into contact with the patient is a breeding ground for pathogens. This is especially true in the optical world, in which the patient's eyes and face touch various instruments and tools.

Every point of contact should be sanitized with an alcohol wipe, following each encounter with a patient. For the optician, this applies primarily to the pupillometer, which is used over and over with every patient. Thoroughly wipe down the nose bumpers, the forehead bar, and any other surface that comes in contact with the patient's face. (For the optometric technician, this extends to the autorefractor, the tonometer, the slit lamp, the phoropter, and any other piece of diagnostic equipment that is used.) The same would apply to a distometer, a PD ruler that was used against the patient's cheek, or any other tool used in the fitting process.

Dispensing Procedures

Determining Best Eyewear Options for Daily Living Needs

This can be summarized in one word: LISTEN. Get the patient talking, and listen to what he or she tells you. The options will suggest themselves.

Do not allow yourself to fall into a "one size fits all" mentality. Every patient is an individual, and so are his or her needs. She may be aware of some of them, but it is the optician's job to think of what she hasn't. An emerging hyperopic presbyope may think she doesn't need that bifocal — that she can get by with readers. But if you ask her how she intends to see who is calling on her cell phone when she's stopped at a red light when driving a car, she might reconsider.

Every patient has a unique set of visual needs. It will be dictated by the things he likes to do in his leisure time, the work he does during the day, or the length and character of his commute. The total picture is the important thing.

Sport- or Hobby-Specific Eyewear

For the person who needs eyewear for a sports activity, the primary goal is always protection. The eyewear should be durable enough for the task and comfortable even if the patient gets hit in the face, and the lenses should be shatterproof.

Furthermore, it can be beneficial to find out whether a patient will be operating in specific lighting situations. For instance, for a patient who usually plays tennis during the daylight, but occasionally plays at night, a pair of photochromatic lenses will do double duty.

The hobbyist who spends all of his time at a bench working with fine tools may benefit from dedicated near-vision glasses, or even glasses with a magnifying loupe, to bring his work into sharp focus with no eyestrain.

The fisherman who spends a lot of time on a boat during the day will appreciate the extra comfort of a blue mirror coating on his sun lenses, to filter out the glare from the sky and water.

Situations in Which a Patient's Intermediate Visual Range Can Be the Primary Concern

When the presbyopic patient finds himself doing an activity that includes little to no distance viewing, only very light reading, and the primary range needed is at arm's length, it may make sense to suggest eyewear that only corrects intermediate vision. A good example is the person who plays the piano for relaxation. Unless he or she is reading a difficult musical score at the same time, intermediate correction alone will prove very useful. This situation may also apply for someone in the kitchen, unless he or she needs to read a lot of recipes.

Lens Options for Use in a Small Office

There is a whole subgenre of progressive-lens offshoots designed for the presbyope and near-presbyope who spends his days in an office environment, looking at a computer either the bulk of his day or all of it. These lenses are collectively called **near-variable-focus** (NVF) lenses, and they can benefit any age patient whose eyes are tired at the end of such a workday.

These lenses, without fail, provide a maximized intermediate range to accommodate a computer monitor. There will be an add at the bottom of the lens (producing the remainder of the near-power not incorporated in the intermediate) to enable the patient to read the occasional fine print, but it will be positioned very low and out of the way.

Some NVF lenses are designed to include a small sliver of distance vision at the very top of the visual field, giving the patient back a smidgen of clarity for across the room. This would never be sufficient for driving home, but it will help him watch the clock until quitting time.

Standards of Frame Measurement

There are five main values that are routinely noted regarding the sizing of a frame. The first four are critical in the lens edging process. All are typically expressed in millimeters.

The **A measurement** is the horizontal distance across one side of the frame, along the lens midline from one inside edge to the opposite inside edge of one eyewire.

The **B measurement** is the vertical distance across the eyewire, down the centerline of one lens.

The **effective diameter (ED)** is defined as the longest distance across the lens, usually on a diagonal.

The **distance between lenses (DBL)** is the same as the bridge measurement, and it is literally the measurement between the furthest nasal points of the lenses.

The fifth measurement is the **temple length**, which is simply the distance from the hinge to the temple tip. Whereas all other frame measurements are consistently metric, temple lengths are still occasionally expressed in inches. This is more common with safety frames, where a 150 mm temple will be listed as 6 inches.

SAE Measurement of 5 Inches into the Correct Number of Millimeters

Most optical measurements will be found in metric units. However, once in a while, the optician may need to convert from SAE measurements into metric, or vice versa. (SAE stands for Society of Automotive Engineers — often, these are simply called English measurements, although in England, the place that originated inches, feet, yards, and miles; they now use the metric system, which originated in France under Napoleon.)

The conversion factor is 25.4 millimeters per inch. Therefore, 5 inches × 25.4 is equal to 127 mm.

Converting a 7 mm Measurement into Centimeters and Then into Meters

The metric system is based on multiples of 10. There are 10 millimeters in a centimeter, 10 centimeters in a decimeter, and 10 decimeters in a meter. Going further, there are 1,000 meters in a kilometer, but this is also a multiple of 10.

Using this simple scheme, it is easy to convert 7 mm into 0.7 cm, or into 0.007 m. The latter is useful in several of the optical formulas, which work in meters, even though most of our measurements are in the much-smaller millimeters. Centimeters are primarily used when discussing a patient's viewing distance, and this measurement will appear on the pupillometer adjustment for taking a near PD.

Measuring Lens Sizing for a Particular Frame

When ordering an edged lens from a lab for a known frame, some type of sizing reference will need to be given, to help ensure a good frame fit upon arrival.

The first of these is an old method called a **Box-o-Graph**, which is simply a grid that the existing lens is held up to. The optician can then record the A, B, and ED of the lens. This is relatively inaccurate, but it does have its uses when the lab will have stock patterns of different sizes. The boxed size of the lens will tell them which pattern to use, in order to match it.

The second method, much more accurate, is called a **C-gauge**. This is a device with a soft tape rule mounted inside it. The lens is placed in the middle of the gauge, and the tape is drawn tight around it, giving a measurement of the lens circumference. The lab can then specify that circumference to be edged, which should match the fit of the existing lens very well.

Measuring Patient's Pupillary Distance

The pupillary distance (PD) is defined as the measurement between pupil centers. It is arguably the most important measurement to be taken during the fitting process, because it will be used in fabrication to ensure that the optical centers of the lenses are positioned directly in front of the patient's eyes.

For generations, the accepted method of taking a PD was by using a simple ruler. With the ruler held close to the patient's eyes, the optician would observe and measure the separation between them. Because locating the middle of a black pupil was difficult, the measurement was often taken at the **limbus** (the outer edge of the iris), from the nasal side of the right eye to the temporal side of the left.

The development of the corneal reflective pupillometer was a major step forward, in that it allowed very accurate measurements (to the half-millimeter), especially when a monocular PD was required. Having the patient peer into the opposite side of the pupillometer, the optician need only line up a vertical crosshair with the reflected spot of light on the patient's cornea.

Situations When Optician Should Measure a Monocular PD vs. a Binocular One

Any fitting of a segmented multifocal generally calls for a binocular PD measurement, simply because of cosmetic concerns. A pair of flat-top bifocals with unequal segment insets will generally be objectionable to the patient. Conversely, for any fitting of a progressive multifocal for which no segment is visible and the accurate positioning of a narrow add corridor is critical, a monocular PD is the accepted norm.

Other than these two scenarios, the decision is up to the optician, based on a number of concerns. Is the precise location of the optical center a concern due to a small optic zone, such as with polycarbonate? Is there a significant right-left difference on the patient, such as after facial trauma? Has horizontal prism been prescribed, which would be affected by displacement of the optical center? These are all situations that demand a monocular PD measurement.

Differentiating Between a Distance PD and a Near PD

Typically, a pair of single-vision glasses are used for correcting distance vision, and so a distance PD would be called for. The exception would be a pair of reading glasses, which call for a near PD. Segmented multifocals are always positioned according to the segments, and so a near PD is required. Progressive multifocals are fitted by the fitting cross just under the distance viewing area, and so they require a distance PD instead. (The old executive multifocals have no discrete segment, and so they are fitted to a distance PD.)

There are two methods for producing a near PD. The most common is to simply measure the distance PD and subtract a standard convergence of 3 or 4 mm from that value. Alternately, the optician can change the viewing range on the pupillometer from infinity to near (usually 40 cm) and remeasure the patient using that setting. The distance and near PDs will usually be given in the format of 65/62 or 63/59.

Measuring the Fitting Height for a Multifocal

In general, the fitting height of a multifocal is taken by dotting the lens with a marking pen, with the patient sitting directly in front of and at eye level with the optician, and then measuring the dot's distance to the bottom eyewire. The following are guidelines only, in what is to be used as reference points.

When measuring the height for a segmented bifocal lens, mark the position of the lower eyelid. For a trifocal, mark the position of the bottom of the pupil. In both cases, the height of the two lenses should usually be matched, for cosmetic reasons, unless the difference is extraordinarily great.

When measuring the height for a progressive lens, the two heights can be independent. Mark the positions of the pupillary centers.

Why Multifocal Fitting Heights Are Not Absolutes

Patients are people, and people have individual needs. With any multifocal height determination, the patient's history should be taken into account, as should her sitting posture and the use she intends to put the glasses to.

For instance, if the patient has previously worn bifocals and is used to them being positioned 4 mm below the lid, then fitting the new lenses at the textbook height of the lower lid will prove to be unacceptably high for her. Ask questions, and listen to the patient's responses.

The patient's posture can be extremely critical, especially when fitting progressive lenses. This is a lens that is easily fit too high, meaning that it interferes with clear distance vision, but it is absolutely useless if fit too low. Because there is no visible line for reference, the patient is relying on you to make the best judgment call as to where his lenses should be positioned for maximum benefit.

Fitting Triangle

All modern eyewear, when fit properly, is anchored at three primary points: the two ears and the bridge of the nose. This is called the fitting triangle, and it must be kept in mind when selecting a frame or dispensing the finished eyewear.

If the frame is too narrow, the temples will push against the side of the head prematurely, rather than anchoring at the ears. This may also cause it not to anchor properly at the nose, as well. If the frame is too wide, the fit will be unstable, and it may be difficult to produce a solid adjustment.

Having given the patient your best advice with these factors in mind, it is the optician's duty to work with the final eyewear choice to produce the best approximation of the fitting-triangle concept.

Producing a Good Cosmetic Adjustment on Patient with Visibly Crooked Face

Any optician is eventually bound to come across a patient with some level of physical asymmetry, whose face simply looks crooked. The frame may have sat perfectly on the bench, but when putting it on the patient, it appears to be bent off-kilter.

The rule of thumb here is that there is a difference between being perfectly straight and looking perfectly straight. The errant feature may be the eyebrows, in which case lining the glasses up with them may solve the problem, making them look straight to the patient and anyone who sees him. The eyes may be at dissimilar levels, in which case bending the frame to center both eyes may be the answer.

In some cases, there may be no perfect solution, and the answer may lie in finding the best compromise between competing considerations.

Properly Fitted Set of Nose Pads

Although nose pads are designed to be self-adjusting, very few patients find that they are comfortable right off the shelf. Most require fine-tuning by the optician either at the fitting or at the point of dispense.

A well-adjusted pair of nose pads will sit on either side of the nose like little feet, squarely on the floor. They are supporting at least one-third of the weight of the glasses, so they must press evenly to distribute that weight properly. Nose pads should never ride along one edge, nor should they poke inward at the bottom or top. And ideally, they should rest on the bony part of the patient's bridge.

In cases in which the bridge is very low or nonexistent (such as frequently seen in Asians), the nose pads may need be rotated nearly 90 degrees, to make contact with the cheekbones. But the same guidelines still apply, in that the pads must distribute the weight as evenly as possible, while providing a firm anchor.

Various Angles to Consider in Nose Pad Adjustment

When moving the nose pads into proper adjustment, there are three angles to consider, corresponding to the three-dimensional motion of the pads as they are adjusted.

The **frontal angle** describes the orientation of the pads as viewed from the front. It mirrors the shape of the nose, widening from top to bottom, so that the bottoms of the pads are further apart than the tops.

The **splay angle** refers to the rotation of the pads as observed from above the frame. The edges closer to the face should be further apart than the edges closer to the frame, again mirroring the shape of the nose.

The **vertical angle** is the pads' position as seen from the side. This will vary anywhere between straight up and down (normal) to a slight forward dive (on a patient with a strong bridge) to a reverse dive toward the patient (when the bridge is weak or absent).

Nose Pad Adjustment to Make Up for Minor Errors in Fitting Height

The ability to adjust nose pads creates a lot of flexibility in fine-tuning the height of a multifocal. If a patient complains of seeing the bifocal too much, it may be positioned slightly too high. Simply increasing the frontal angle, bringing the nose pads slightly further apart, will lower the bifocal height a millimeter or two and may solve the problem. Likewise, a patient who feels the bifocal is just a bit too low may be satisfied by decreasing the frontal angle, bringing the nose pads closer together and raising the height a millimeter or two.

Proper Adjustment of Skull-Fit Temples

Temples that are designed to curve gently over the ear and downward behind it are referred to as skull-fit temples.

Manufacturers once made frames with multiple temple lengths to choose from, but most have now fallen into supplying a standard temple length and nothing else. It then becomes the optician's job to help the patient select a frame with a usable temple length and to adjust it properly before the patient leaves with the glasses.

A properly fit skull temple will remain straight all the way back to the top of the ear, where it will gently curve over and follow the contour of the back of the ear. It should not press against the ear, but it should rest gently against the side of the head. Likewise, it should not press hard against the mastoid bone, behind the ear. Either scenario will cause the patient discomfort, or this can cause the temple to pop up rather than staying properly seated.

Steps to Take When Frame Feels Tight, but Glasses Still Slide Down

This problem usually boils down to the temples making contact with the patient's head too far in front of the ears. On top of causing the glasses to slide downward, this can eventually leave permanent marks on the sides of the patient's head.

To correct the problem, first open up the frame by widening the angle of the temples at the end pieces. Then gently curve the ends of the temples back toward the ears. Check for fit, making sure not to create too much space between the temple and the side of the head, but just enough to cause the temples to touch down right at the ear. Readjust the temple tips for comfort, if necessary.

Correcting a Frame that Appears Too High on One Side

A frame that appears too high on the right side can be corrected by angling the right temple upward, or the left temple downward. Conversely, a frame that appears too high on the left side can be corrected by angling the left temple upward or the right temple downward.

The choice of which side to angle up or down will be determined by the existing pantoscopic tilt because this adjustment will change it in one direction or the other; i.e., angling either temple downward may solve the height problem but will increase the pantoscopic tilt at the same time. Choose whichever direction will leave the tilt in an acceptable position.

Alternatives to Skull-Fit Temples

Although they are much less common, there are other temples available besides skull-fit. Their availability is strictly limited to a handful of frames by certain manufacturers.

An older style that was once much more prevalent is the **cable temple**. This is a temple with a flexible end that curls around the ear. Some patients were fiercely loyal to this design, but despite their wails of protest, most manufacturers have discontinued them entirely. Some children's frames may still be found with this feature, because it can be invaluable in keeping glasses on an infant or toddler.

A newer temple style is called the **occipital-fit temple**. This design does not curve around the ear at all but goes straight back and curves slightly around the head (in the occipital area of the skull, hence the name). These temple styles are found mainly in sporty eyewear and certain sunglasses, and they are often sought out by patients who are after a particular look (including the ability to prop the sunglasses on top of the head), rather than a practical fit.

Frame Tilt

A line drawn from the average person's brow to his cheek will tend inward from the vertical by about 5–10 degrees. The typical frame is designed to mimic this fact, by being angled inward at the bottom by the same amount. This normal inward angling of the frame is referred to as pantoscopic tilt. In addition to providing a pleasing appearance, this angle produces more natural vision below the line of sight. (The reverse, outward angling at the bottom, is called **retroscopic tilt**, and it is generally to be avoided.)

A frame's pantoscopic tilt can be adjusted by angling the temples up or down. Angling them downward will increase pantoscopic tilt, whereas angling upward will reduce it. The average patient feels most comfortable with a small amount of pantoscopic tilt. Too little of it (or retroscopic tilt) will make the floor look distorted and produce a visual gap below the glasses, whereas too much of it will make it hard for a presbyope to read with his multifocals, because the near zone appears too close to his cheek.

Face-Form

The typical frame is designed to curve gently across the front, wrapping slightly around the curvature of the average patient's face. This curvature is called face-form, and it is comfortable to the patient in small amounts. Increasing face-form too much can result in distorted vision and patient discomfort.

Certain sport and sunglass frames are manufactured with intentionally steep face-form, either to maximize eye protection, to increase sun protection, or simply to achieve a sporty look. When a sunglass is made this way, it is often referred to simply as a wrapped frame, and often a steeper-than-normal base curve must be used. In these cases, the patient must be prepared to acclimate himself to the resulting alterations in his vision.

Effect of Vertex Distance on Frame Selection and Adjustment

When the optometrist refracts the patient, he does so with the phoropter a specific, fixed distance from the eyes, typically about 15 mm. This is called his vertex distance. Depending on frame fit, this may or may not be the same as the final distance to the patient's lenses. In higher prescriptions, a small variation will alter the effective prescription for the patient, unless a compensated lens is ordered.

To reduce these effects, steer these patients toward frames that will fit their bridges snugly and closely, once adjusted. A pair of glasses that slides around excessively can actually change the prescription as the patient sees it.

Significance of Face-Form, Tilt, and Vertex in Digital Lens Fitting

The free-form revolution in lens manufacturing has opened up the possibilities for patient-by-patient customization of the final product. The most cutting-edge progressive lens technology allows the dispenser to take into account all aspects of the individual frame fit, in order to achieve one-of-a-kind optics for each patient, maximizing every twitch of the eye muscles into a better visual experience.

When ordering such lenses, the lab will ask for additional parameters such as tilt, wrap, and vertex as part of the lens design process. Therefore, when ordering such lenses, it is critical to make sure a complete and accurate frame adjustment is done as part of the initial fitting so as to ensure that those values do not change at the final dispense.

Most Important Thing When Sitting Down with Patient for Fitting

When beginning the process of fitting a patient with any eyewear, the most important thing the optician can do is to position himself directly in front of the patient and at the same eye level. This will produce the most accurate PD and height measurements and ensure that the patient's finished eyewear will be as usable as possible.

The optician should also make sure that the patient is relaxed and comfortable, which will ensure that she is fully cooperative in the measuring process. Her posture should be natural for her, so that the finished eyewear will function well in that position.

Concerns When Fitting Children with Eyewear

Children can be tricky to fit, and the younger they are, the more of a challenge they can be. For one thing, their attention span will be very short, so although the optician needs accurate measurements, he must often get them quickly or not at all.

It is always helpful to address the child on his own level, getting and holding his attention in whatever way necessary. Make a game out of the pupillometer, as you cause one image to vanish while the other one magically appears. In very young children, you may have to abandon the pupillometer and use a ruler instead if they can't keep their eyes on the target long enough for a reading or if they simply are too young to understand.

Frame choice for a very young child can be a challenge because it is often a problem keeping the eyewear on their face. Cable temples can solve this problem, but at the expense of dangerous nose pads. Plastic frames can sometimes be adjusted to grip the ear snugly, but the best alternative is a soft frame with an elastic strap to hold it in place.

Critical Concerns When Dispensing Eyewear

There are three things the new glasses must adhere to, when dispensing them to the patient: looking good, feeling good, and being medically correct.

Looking good refers to the overall balanced and level appearance of the glasses on the patient, making the best of her (and your) choice of frame and lenses.

Feeling good refers to the overall comfort of the glasses as the patient wears them. The glasses should fit solidly but not be pinching, pulling, or poking the patient anywhere. A proper adjustment will go a long way toward addressing both of these first two elements, but the patient should also be free from any excessive eyestrain or visual discomfort.

A medically correct prescription should have been determined before the patient arrives, but the ability of the glasses to correct and improve on her vision should be demonstrated at the dispensing table.

Verifying Patient's Vision with New Eyewear

A patient can verify the effectiveness of a new pair of single-vision glasses by simply being asked to observe what is around him. For myopic prescriptions that have just increased, ask the patient to focus on the leaves in the trees outside the window or to read a sign across the street that he couldn't before. For hyperopes, have the patient look at a computer screen or some reading material that was previously giving him a hard time. If a Snellen chart is on hand, ask the patient to read from it.

For the multifocal patient, the above can be applied to his distance vision, but the optician should go a step further and verify the near vision with a reading card. Make sure the patient is able to read any fine print that may have been eluding him previously.

Important Elements in Patient Education at Point of Dispense

First and foremost, it is important to remind the patient that any new pair of glasses, even when there was no change in the Rx, can take some getting used to. Nose pads will be pressing in new places, temples are not going to fit identically to the old ones, and even the vision might seem slightly different due to any number of minor changes in lens material or fit of the frame front.

If there has been an Rx change, the patient may feel a bit disoriented or her vision may be a bit unsettling at first. Stronger minus lenses will make the ground seem to curve upward at her, and stronger plus lenses will shift it backward toward her feet, and either may cause her to stumble at first, if she is not mindful. New progressive wearers need to be cautious of this same thing, because that entire half of his visual field will now appear out of focus unless she tilts her face down to look directly at it. In extreme cases, it can be advisable to suggest that the patient wear the old glasses home, wait until the next morning, and put the new glasses on right after waking up.

Concerns to Discuss with Patient Regarding Care of Lenses with Specific Features

Antireflective coatings (even the best ones) require some special precautions. For one, they should always be cleaned with a soft cloth, and harsh chemicals should always be avoided. For another, their biggest enemy is high heat, and the patient should be cautioned against leaving them in a hot car, especially in the overhead bins that carmakers have been placing there for that specific purpose. (This is the absolute hottest point in the car.)

Mirror-coated lenses are even more delicate, although they are more susceptible to abrasion than heat. No coated lenses should ever be laid facedown on a surface. Mirror coatings are especially unforgiving of this, and the results will be immediate and very obvious. More than with any other eyewear, the rule of thumb here should be on your face, or in the case.

Glass photochromatic lenses will not change color all the way immediately, but they must be broken in by exposing them to a great deal of direct sunlight, such as on a window ledge. Plastic photochromatics will change immediately, but they may get sluggish in hot weather and respond to a boost by putting them in the freezer.

Laws, Regulations, and Standards

ANSI

The American National Standards Institute (ANSI) is the organization that sets commercial and industrial standards for a wide variety of products and business activities, including those of the eye care industry. The section that deals with eyewear is numbered Z80.1, and because its latest revision happened in 2015, it is commonly referred to as ANSI Z80.1-2015.

ANSI has no formal authority to enforce these standards, which are left up to the individual practitioners to follow. The only exception to this is the subsection that deals with industrial-safety eyewear, which has been officially adopted by the Occupational Safety and Health Administration.

General Rules That Apply to Eyewear Tolerances

In general terms, eyewear tolerances try to take into account human error. Perfection would be ideal, but this is not always attainable. Thus, there is a margin of error established for all values observed in a finalized pair of eyewear.

With lens powers, the tolerances widen with increased power, simply because smaller errors become unnoticeable against the bigger picture. With cylinder axis, the exact opposite is true, because the effect of an off-axis lens increases so dramatically as the cylinder gets stronger. With prismatic imbalance, the tolerances remain nearly the same across all powers, with only a slight bit more wiggle room above a certain power... again, because the effect of prismatic error on the patient is so profound.

Frequently Referenced Standards That Apply to Dress Eyewear

No optician is expected to memorize Z80.1 in its entirety, but certain elements that are very frequently used should become committed to memory.

Sphere powers:	± 0.13D, up to ± 6.50 D
	± 2%, above 6.50 D
Cylinder powers:	± 0.13 D, up to 2.00 D
	± 0.15 D, from 2.00 to 4.50 D
	± 4%, above 4.50 D
Cylinder axis:	± 14, up to 0.25 D
	± 7, from 0.37 to 0.50 D
	± 5, from 0.62 to 0.75 D
	± 3, from 0.87 to 1.50 D
	± 2, above 1.50 D
Horizontal prism:	0.67 D, from plano to ± 2.75 D
	< 2.5 mm from PD, above 2.75 D
Vertical prism:	0.33D, from plano to ± 3.375 D
	< 1.0 mm from PRP*, above 3.375 D

(*PRP = prism reference point, usually the PD or the OC.)

Special Considerations in Fabrication and Dispensing of Industrial Safety Eyewear

The ANSI subsection that deals with safety eyewear is numbered Z87.1. When assembling a pair of safety eyewear, any frame materials must be clearly marked with this designation, or it is not acceptable. Any lenses must be monogrammed with the lab's unique identifier.

Safety eyewear falls under one of two designations: basic impact or high impact. The ballistic testing is more stringent for the second category. For basic impact, the finished lens must survive a drop-ball test in which a 1-inch steel ball is dropped from a height of 50 inches. High impact calls for a 1/4-inch steel ball to be fired at the lens at 150 ft/sec, and the lens monogram will have a + after the lab's insignia. Basic impact eyewear must be dispensed with a disclaimer, clearly stating that it is not high impact.

Special Treatment That Glass Lenses Must Receive Prior to Dispensing

Besides the special hardening techniques that must be performed after edging a glass lens, ANSI standards require that prior to mounting in the frame, it must survive a drop-ball test in which a 5/8-inch steel ball is dropped from a height of 50 inches. The results of this pass/fail test must be documented and kept in the patient's file for a period of three years.

ASTM

The American Society for Testing Materials (ASTM) is the organization that is responsible for standards in sports-related products. Section F803 of their rulings is the area that pertains to protective eyewear used in sports.

All sport-protective eyewear should be made with polycarbonate or Trivex lenses with a minimum center thickness of 2 mm. Frame manufacturers perform stringent impact testing as part of the manufacturing process, using stock plano lenses. Those who adhere to the ASTM standards will always indicate this on the frame with the designation ASTM F803.

NOCE Practice Test

Want to take this practice test in an online interactive format?
Check out the bonus page, which includes interactive practice questions and much more:
https://www.mometrix.com/bonus948/noce

1. What strength is a lens measured in?

a. Microns
b. Add powers
c. Diopters
d. Prisms

2. What will light rays passing through a "plus" lens always do?

a. Diverge
b. Converge
c. Cohere
d. Disperse

3. What is the principal action on light passing from one medium into another of different density called?

a. Displacement
b. Convergence
c. Diffraction
d. Refraction

4. What range of UV light is typically responsible for sunburns?

a. 10 nanometers to 100 nanometers
b. 320 nanometers to 400 nanometers
c. 100 nanometers to 290 nanometers
d. 290 nanometers to 320 nanometers

5. What is the measure of how far it takes a lens to bring light to a point?

a. Focal length
b. Major axis
c. Power
d. Base curve

6. What is the spacing between the surface of the eye and the inside surface of a corrective lens known as?

a. Sagittal depth
b. Fitting cross
c. Seg drop
d. Vertex distance

7. What element of an eyeglass prescription is a measure of the patient's myopia or hyperopia?

a. Cylinder
b. Axis
c. Sphere
d. Add power

8. What are the two modern forms in which a prescription may be written?

a. Plus-cylinder and minus-cylinder
b. Cross-cylinder and plus-cylinder
c. Spherical and aspherical
d. Base curve and cross curve

9. A prescription of OD -0.25, OS Plano, add $+1.75$ is primarily indicating what type of refractive error?

a. Hyperopia
b. Presbyopia
c. Stigmatism
d. Nystagmus

10. A prescription for a patient with astigmatism will contain which of the following elements?

a. Cylinder and sphere
b. Axis and add power
c. Cylinder and axis
d. Cylinder and prism

11. A prescription of OD $+1.00$ -0.50 X 31 OS $+1.75$ -1.25 X 168 is an example of what kind of prescription?

a. Spherocylindrical
b. Myopic
c. Aspheric
d. Anisometropic

12. A prescription is written as follows: OD -1.25 $+1.75$ X 110. What transposed prescription would be written on the lab order?

a. −3.00 −1.75 X 10
b. +0.50 −1.75 X 110
c. Plano +1.75 X 30
d. +0.50 −1.75 X 20

13. If a patient insists on glasses for "near-vision only," which would be the correctly transposed numbers to order the following OU prescription: -0.75 $+2.50$ X 11 add $+1.25$?

a. +1.75 −2.50 X 101
b. +3.00 −2.50 X 101
c. +0.50 +2.50 X 101
d. +3.00 +2.50 X 11

14. One of the early solutions for extreme hyperopia was a type of lens with a very steep curvature in a small central portion, surrounded by a flat carrier edge. This was known as what type of lens?

a. Myodisc
b. Meniscus
c. Lenticular
d. Corrected-curve

15. What is a lens with a single curvature on the front and two curvatures on the back called?

a. Cylindrical
b. Aphakic
c. Aspheric
d. Toric

16. What is the power of a corrective lens referred to as when calculated purely from its measurable curvatures?

a. Effective power
b. Surface power
c. Vertex power
d. Corrected power

17. What is the average refractive index of a polycarbonate lens?

a. 1.56
b. 1.60
c. 1.58
d. 1.67

18. What is the measurement of optical clarity of a lens called?

a. Reflectance
b. Transmittance
c. Snellen equivalent
d. Abbe value

19. What is the spherical equivalent of the following prescription: −2.25 +3.50 X 171?

a. −0.50
b. −2.25
c. +0.50
d. +1.25

20. Given the prescription +1.00 −2.00 X 135, what is the effective power in the 90th meridian?

a. −1.00
b. −3.00
c. Plano
d. +1.00

21. A prescription of +1.75 −2.75 X 153 would be written in what way by an ophthalmologist?

a. +4.50 +2.75 X 63
b. −1.00 +2.75 X 63
c. −1.00 +2.75 X 153
d. −2.75 +1.75 X 153

22. A +4.00 lens intended to be positioned at a PD of 30 mm was actually manufactured at 33 mm. What is the amount of prism induced by this error?

a. 12 diopters
b. 0.75 diopters
c. 1.33 diopters
d. 1.2 diopters

23. Vertical imbalance error is always read at the _____ lens in the 90th meridian.

a. more minus
b. more plus
c. weaker
d. stronger

24. What is the dioptric power of a lens with a focal length of 400 mm?

a. +2.50
b. −2.50
c. +4.00
d. +0.25

25. A patient is refracted at 13 mm with a prescription of +12. 00 OU, but it is found that the frame she selected will hold the lenses at a distance of 18 mm from her eyes. What prescription should the optician order to compensate for this discrepancy?

a. +12.77
b. +13.25
c. +10.77
d. +11.23

26. What kind of lens has powers that vary smoothly as the viewing angle is raised and lowered?

a. Trifocal lens
b. Progressive lens
c. Aniseikonic lens
d. Intra-ocular lens

27. Which of the following is true regarding full-seg or "executive" bifocals?

a. They are popular with younger presbyopes.
b. They are easy to manufacture in a wide variety of prescriptions.
c. They have the widest near field of view of any bifocal.
d. They incorporate the latest technological advances.

28. Which of the following multifocal styles will produce the least amount of image jump for the patient?

a. Progressive
b. Round-seg
c. Flat-top
d. Blended

29. The inlaid segment in a glass bifocal is made of what material?

a. Didydium glass
b. Lead glass
c. Crown glass
d. Flint glass

30. What would be the best choice of lens for a presbyopic patient who relies heavily on his glasses at work for near vision in more than one location at a time?

a. Progressives
b. Double-D bifocals
c. Near-vision only
d. Photochromatic lenses

31. Which type of multifocal will give the patient the maximum room in the intermediate visual zone?

a. 8x35 trifocals
b. CRT lenses
c. 7x28 trifocals
d. NVF lenses

32. Which of the following is NOT true of Trivex lenses?

a. They are the thinnest and lightest lens alternative.
b. They are the most impact-resistant lenses available.
c. They have an optical clarity roughly equal to that of glass.
d. They tend to be more expensive to produce.

33. Which lens material offers the best resistance to corrosive chemicals?

a. CR-39
b. Trivex
c. Polycarbonate
d. Crown glass

34. A 15-year-old patient is selecting glasses. The prescription is as follows: OD -3.75 -1.50 X 18, OS -4.25 -0.75 X 167. It has been stated that he is on a tight budget. What is the best choice of lens material for this patient?

a. Trivex
b. 1.67 high-index
c. Polycarbonate
d. Spectralite

35. What is the measure of a lens material's ability to bend light?

a. Angle of incidence
b. Index of refraction
c. Abbe value
d. Visual field

36. A patient comes to you with a high prescription, OD -9.25, OS -9.50. The patient is willing to pay for the thinnest lens available but makes it known that clear vision is important. What lens material should this patient be wearing?

a. High-index 1.60
b. Spectralite
c. High-index 1.71
d. High-index 1.67

37. Which of the following eye conditions will most likely require the use of prism in the prescription?

a. Astigmatism
b. Hyperopia
c. Diplopia
d. Presbyopia

38. A ray of light passing through a prism is bent toward the _____.

a. apex.
b. base.
c. center.
d. temporal.

39. What amount of decentration, and in which direction, will induce 2 diopters of base-in prism for a -3.75 lens?

a. 0.53 mm nasally
b. 1.87 mm temporally
c. 5.33 mm nasally
d. 5.33 mm temporally

40. Which phrase best describes the use of prism to correct imbalance at the reading level due to anisometropia?

a. Base-down prism applied to the upper portion of the most-minus lens
b. Base-up prism applied to the lower portion of the most-minus lens
c. Base-up prism applied to the upper portion of the most-plus lens
d. Base-in prism applied to the lower portion of the most-minus lens

41. What amount of unwanted vertical prism error is acceptable in the finished eyewear for a patient wearing an Rx of OD -4.25 -0.75 X 173, OS -4.50 SPH?

a. 1/3 diopter as measured at the left lens
b. 2 mm as measured at the left lens
c. 2/3 diopter as measured at the left lens
d. 1/3 diopter as measured at the right lens

42. What is a 1.5 diopter horizontal prism for a patient with a mild esophoria known as?

a. Compound
b. Induced
c. Palliative
d. Slab-off

43. The largest chamber of the eye's interior structure holds which bodily fluid?

a. Aqueous humor
b. Lymphatic fluid
c. Plasma
d. Vitreous humor

44. What is the primary refracting body of the eye?

a. Crystalline lens
b. Optic disk
c. Cornea
d. Medial canthus

45. Which elements of the retina are specifically responsible for helping us see in color?

a. Rods
b. Cones
c. Stroma
d. Fovea

46. Tears are typically removed from the eye by the _______.

a. lateral canthus.
b. lacrimal puncta.
c. meibomian glands.
d. superior rectus.

47. What refractive condition results from one eye requiring a much-stronger lens than the other eye?

a. Myopia
b. Emmetropia
c. Astigmatism
d. Anisometropia

48. The layperson will often describe him- or herself as "farsighted." What condition is the person suffering from?

a. Hyperopia
b. Presbyopia
c. Myopia
d. Xerostomia

49. In the condition known as myopia, at which point in the eye do the light rays naturally come to focus?

a. At the fovea
b. Behind the retina
c. In front of the retina
d. At the optic disk

50. If a patient's eye brings some of the light to focus in front of the retina, and some of it behind the retina, he or she is said to have which condition?

a. Hyperopic astigmatism
b. Compound myopic astigmatism
c. Regular astigmatism
d. Mixed astigmatism

51. A 42-year-old patient presents to you complaining of her eyes being tired at the end of a day of staring at a computer screen, and the patient is unable to read the paper after dinner. What is the most likely problem?

a. Hyperopia
b. Presbyopia
c. Nystagmus
d. Phthisis

52. What is the most commonly used metal found in eyeglass frames?

a. Gold
b. Steel
c. Monel
d. Aluminum

53. What is a frame with a solid bar above the lenses and a nylon filament below them known as?

a. Rimless
b. Nylon
c. 3-piece
d. Semi-rimless

54. What is the most important thing to avoid when working with a frame made of Optyl?

a. Making any adjustments as the material cools
b. Heating the frame in any way
c. Getting the frame wet
d. Stretching the frame beyond its shape and size

55. Which of the following is NOT a property of cellulose acetate frames?

a. It is very durable.
b. It is hypoallergenic.
c. It takes heat very well.
d. Its color fades over time.

56. What lens material possesses the highest impact resistance?

a. Glass
b. Trivex
c. CR-39
d. Polycarbonate

57. Progressive-addition lenses excel in all but which of the following characteristics?

a. Maximum usable visual field
b. Smooth transition from distance to near vision
c. Availability in a variety of materials
d. Designed for a variety of uses

58. What is a progressive-style lens configured for a heavy computer user that offers no area for distance vision called?

a. Single-vision
b. CRT
c. Near variable focus
d. Open-angle

59. The upper ribbon in a typical trifocal lens is equal to which value in the patient's prescription?

a. Sphere power divided by two
b. One-half the prescribed add power
c. Twice the prescribed add power
d. One-third the prescribed cylinder power

60. Polarization in a sunglass lens is generally achieved in what manner?

a. A very dark lens tint
b. An impregnated light filter
c. A laminate on the surface
d. A photochromatic tint

61. Which of the following lens coatings or treatments will be beneficial to the most patients?

a. U-V protection
b. Photochromatic tint
c. Mirror coating
d. Anti-reflective coating

62. Which of the following is a true statement regarding photochromatic lenses?

a. They provide a variable tint under differing lighting situations.
b. They are available in every lens design and material.
c. They can replace a separate pair of sunglasses.
d. They are perfect for every patient.

63. All of the following are characteristics of a CR-39 lens EXCEPT

a. crisp optics.
b. shatter resistance.
c. lightweight.
d. blocking 50% of the UV.

64. A patient with a prescription of OD −1.00 −3.75 X 47, OS −0.75 −4.00 X 129 will have lenses that tend to be thickest at what point?

a. Upper nasal corner
b. Bottom edge
c. Lower temporal corner
d. Upper temporal corner

65. The prescription reads +1.50 Sphere, Add +2.50 OU, and the patient has indicated that he or she wants "no-line bifocals." Which frame type will be the most problematic and best avoided?

a. Zyl
b. Drilled rimless
c. Semi-rimless
d. Full-rim metal

66. Which frame and bridge style will distribute the weight of the glasses most evenly?

a. Nose pads
b. Padless metal bridge
c. Keyhole bridge
d. Saddle bridge

67. Given the prescription +2.50 −3.00 X 86, and a standard-fit frame, what ideal base curvature would the optician select when placing the lab order?

a. +5.25
b. +7.25
c. +6.25
d. +4.25

68. What is an example of when a polarized lens may not be the right choice for the patient?

a. The patient does a lot of daytime driving.
b. The patient is a fisherman.
c. The patient needs to read digital displays while in bright sun.
d. The patient spends time at the beach.

69. In which of the following situations will a photochromatic lens typically be the least effective?

a. Driving a car
b. Frequently stepping outdoors
c. Playing sports
d. Going to a baseball game

70. A patient tells you she is having trouble with nighttime driving. Asking further, you discover that the unattenuated glare from headlights on rainy roads is the worst problem. Which product would most likely solve this dilemma?

a. A light-yellow tint
b. A polarized lens
c. A mirror coating
d. An anti-reflective coating

71. You are faced with a 35-year-old patient who is a computer programmer. She is experiencing tired eyes by the end of her day, but she and the doctor agree that she is too young for a bifocal. What may be a good solution for her situation?

a. A progressive lens with the lowest add power, which you append to the prescription
b. A new pair of single-vision lenses
c. An anti-fatigue lens
d. A pair of over-the-counter readers

72. A 48-year-old patient who is a house painter complains that he can't see clearly to paint under eaves. You determine that a double-D occupational bifocal will help. What extra step must you take prior to ordering the lenses?

a. Check the insurance for second-pair coverage.
b. Find the two working distances he most commonly needs.
c. Decide the way he will wear the frame.
d. Ask what color of paint he uses most often.

73. A first-time presbyope wants progressive lenses, and she has chosen a frame for the new glasses. What is the first consideration in the lens choice you will help her make?

a. A price she can easily afford
b. The brand name of the lens
c. The color of his photochromatic tint
d. A corridor length that will fit easily within the frame

74. An elderly patient with full aphakia presents you with a prescription of OD +14.25 −1.25 X 003, OS +15.00 −0.75 X 171, add +3.50. What should be the first lens option that comes to mind?

a. Compensated powers
b. Progressives
c. Aspherics
d. Anti-reflective coating

75. At what location on a progressive-addition lens will prescribed prism be verified?

a. At the fitting cross
b. At the manufacturer's reference point
c. In the center of the distance circle
d. At the top of the add circle

76. When determining the presence and degree of unwanted vertical imbalance in a completed pair of single-vision eyewear, it is important to begin with the ______ lens.

a. weaker
b. more minus
c. more plus
d. stronger

77. A completed pair of flat-top bifocals has been received from the lab, is being inspected by the optician, and appears questionable in a few ways. Which problem will most likely be of greatest concern to the patient?

a. Crooked segments
b. 11-degree axis error
c. 0.18D power error
d. Wrong A-R coating

78. What is the process of "truing" a frame prior to dispensing it?

a. Pre-adjustment
b. Bench alignment
c. Pantoscopic tilt
d. Face-form

79. Verification of any photochromatic properties of the completed eyewear can be done using what means?

a. Polariscope
b. Lensometer
c. Direct observation
d. Photometer

80. A completed pair of eyewear arrives from the lab. What is the first thing the optician should take note of?

a. The prescription is accurate
b. The lens style is correct
c. The lens tint matches the order
d. The lenses are in the proper frame

81. What is the part of the lensometer that is used to determine the diopters of a lens known as?

a. Frame table
b. Axis wheel
c. Power drum
d. Spotting pins

82. When a single image in the lensometer comes into focus at two different powers, this indicates the presence of what prescription element?

a. Cylinder
b. Add power
c. Prism
d. Aberration

83. When reading add powers on a segmented multifocal, it is suggested to pay attention to what detail?

a. The power may not match the written prescription.
b. The segments may not be aligned.
c. The lenses may scratch easily.
d. The power should be read from the back.

84. What device may be used to determine the surface curvature of a lens?

a. Leap blocker
b. Spherometer
c. Polariscope
d. Protractor

85. When beginning to read lens powers on a lensometer, after centering the image in the reticle, what is the next step?

a. Rotate the axis wheel by 90 degrees.
b. Rotate the power drum until the image comes into focus.
c. Rotate the power drum all the way toward the plus end.
d. Turn the prism compensator until the image is 2 diopters off center.

86. On an older lensometer, the reading of extremely strong prism may require the use of what device?

a. Radius gauge
b. Altimeter
c. Auxiliary prism ring
d. Sagitta gauge

87. When is it necessary to know the drop and inset of a flat-top bifocal?

a. When verifying prescribed prism
b. When ordering for a sensitive patient
c. When measuring a patient's fitting height
d. When reading the add power

88. When reading the prescribed power of a progressive-addition lens, where is it verified?

a. Anywhere in the upper half of the lens
b. At the manufacturer's reference point
c. In the center of the power corridor
d. In the center of the distance circle

89. Which is a correct part of the verification process with any completed eyewear?

a. After reading the first lens, move the frame table out of the way before placing the opposite lens at the eyepiece.
b. After reading the first lens, unclamp it, and leave the frame table in place, while centering the opposite lens at the eyepiece.
c. After reading the right lens, unclamp it, and clamp the left lens into place, ignoring the frame table altogether
d. After reading the right lens, assume that the left lens will also be acceptable.

90. What is the first thing to do when beginning the verification of any eyewear at a lensometer?

a. Dial in the sphere power of the OD lens.
b. Switch the power off and then back on.
c. Focus the eyepiece.
d. Spin the axis wheel 180 degrees.

91. What is the proper way to take a patient's near PD using a pupilometer?

a. Line up the crosshairs at the nasal limbus, and record the reading.
b. With the instrument set to infinity, line up the crosshairs with the centers of the corneas, and subtract 3 from the reading.
c. Ask the patient if he or she happens to know his or her PD, and subtract 5 from the answer.
d. With the instrument set to 35 cm, line up the crosshairs with the centers of the corneas, and record the reading.

92. What instrument is used to determine the finished thickness of a lens?

a. Lens caliper
b. Lens clock
c. Sagitta gauge
d. C-gauge

93. What is the function of a polariscope?

a. To read the base curve of a lens
b. To locate manufacturers' markings on a progressive lens
c. To observe stress patterns within a lens
d. To tell if a lens is polarized

94. A patient needs a single lens replaced in a frame that he cannot give up to send to the lab. The frame model is known to the lab, but you are concerned with the new lens being the correct size when it arrives. What small piece of equipment will solve the problem?

a. Lens washer
b. C-gauge
c. Pattern cutter
d. Lens caliper

95. What tool would be best used to take a patient's vertex measurement?

a. Ruler
b. Distometer
c. Lens clock
d. Lens caliper

96. What precaution should be taken when using a frame warmer to adjust any eyewear with anti-reflective-coated lenses?

a. None, the entire frame can be heated without concern.
b. Only the temple tips should be heated.
c. Heat may be applied to the corners of the frame in moderation.
d. The lenses should be removed prior to any heating of the frame.

97. An otherwise properly adjusted lensometer appears to be reading all powers off by 0.25 in the plus direction. How might this small error be easily corrected?

a. Taping a −0.25D test lens to the eyepiece
b. Turning the lamp brightness to a lower level
c. Adjusting the pointer next to the power drum
d. Simply subtracting 0.25 from every prescription you verify

98. What simple procedure will keep any ophthalmic instrument in better working order?

a. Keeping it covered while not in use
b. Cleaning the entire instrument with alcohol daily
c. Not allowing the patients to touch it
d. Not allowing children loose in the office

99. While verifying work at the lensometer, the optician notes that the higher the lens power, the more inaccurate the reading seems to grow. The error is only in one direction; that is, high-minus lenses seem to read higher minus than they should, whereas higher pluses read weaker than they should. Where does the problem lie?

a. The power drum is warped.
b. The lab is experiencing a quality problem.
c. The eyepiece needs to be adjusted.
d. The lens stop needs to be adjusted.

100. What is a good practice to adopt with instruments that come into contact with patients?

a. Sanitize points of contact daily.
b. Sanitize points of contact after each patient.
c. Pretreat points of contact with germicidal chemicals.
d. Cover all points of contact with disposable paper.

101. A patient tells you that she plays tennis and has ruined a pair or two of glasses by getting them knocked off while playing. Further questions reveal that she usually plays in the daytime but occasionally at night. What solution suggests itself for this patient?

a. Contact lenses
b. A rugged pair of safety glasses with an elastic strap
c. A comfortable pair of sports eyewear with photochromatic lenses
d. Going without his glasses while playing tennis

102. What visual range(s) is(are) most critical for the presbyopic patient who plays piano for relaxation and only plays by ear?

a. Intermediate vision
b. Near vision
c. Near and intermediate vision
d. Distance vision

103. Bob is 57 and works in shipping and receiving. He spends about half his day entering data into a computer, but the other half, he walks about a warehouse, where he is required to locate specifically labeled bins and storage compartments that are often above eye level. He is not so concerned about the look of his glasses as he is with how well they work in this demanding environment. What lens would you suggest for Bob?

a. Progressives
b. Flat-top bifocals
c. NVF lenses
d. CRT trifocals

104. Carl is a 49-year-old electrician. He spends his day in a combination of reading diagrams and peering up into breaker boxes to follow wiring and read small labels. What type of lens would suit him best at work?

a. Progressives
b. Near-vision only
c. Double-D bifocals
d. Standard trifocals

105. Lucy is a computer programmer and has been wearing progressives since her late 30s because of all the time she spends at the screen. Lately, however, she is finding that the intermediate portion of the corridor is not enough, and it is tiring her eyes before the end of the day. What might be a good choice for her?

a. Near-vision only
b. Intermediate-vision only
c. Occupational bifocals
d. NVF lenses

106. What is the accepted starting point for measuring the fitting height of a standard trifocal lens?

a. Bottom of the pupil
b. Center of the pupil
c. Lower eyelid
d. Lower limbus

107. A patient wearing a metal frame complains that the reading area seems "too high" and often in the way. Upon inspection, you note that the frame front is angled beyond vertical so that the bottom of his frame is further from his face than the top. What adjustment should you make to correct this problem?

a. Increase retroscopic tilt
b. Increase pantoscopic tilt
c. Add face form
d. Increase nose pad splay angle

108. What tool(s) would you use to adjust a metal frame so that the bottom sits closer to the patient's cheek?

a. Nose pad pliers
b. Half-round and axis pliers
c. Numont and angling pliers
d. Compression pliers

109. Which of the following situations definitely requires the measuring of an optical center height?

a. Fitting a pair of trifocal lenses
b. Replacing a single bifocal lens
c. Fitting a pair of single-vision polycarbonate lenses
d. Fitting a pair of progressive lenses

110. When verifying a finished pair of progressive-addition lenses at the lensometer, you have identified the stronger lens as your starting point. What are the next steps to take and why?

a. Read the distance powers in the distance circle, noting any deviations that may be outside of tolerances, then remove the glasses from the lensometer and measure PDs and heights.
b. Read the distance powers in the distance circle, read the add powers, noting any deviations that may be outside of tolerances, then remove the glasses and measure PDs and heights.
c. Center the MRPs, reading the powers and noting any deviations that may be outside of tolerances, then remove the glasses and measure PDs and heights
d. Center the MRPs, noting any deviation on the weaker lens that may constitute vertical imbalance, then read the distance and near powers in the circles, noting any deviations outside of tolerances, and finally remove the glasses and measure PDs and heights.

111. A pair of single-vision glasses has arrived from the lab, and you are verifying it at the lensometer. The prescription is OD -4.00 -0.25 X 179, OS -4.75 Sph, and the specified PDs are 32/33. The power parameters are all within tolerance, but when spotting the centers and measuring the PDs, you find that the right lens is at 29 and the left is at 32. Which lens(es) must be remade, and what amount of unwanted prism was induced in that lens?

a. OS, 4.75D prism
b. OS, 0.475D prism
c. OD, 1.2D prism
d. Both OD and OS, 1.2D and 0.475D prism

112. When measuring the PD of a patient who will be wearing progressive lenses, what is the best method to use?

a. Monocular PD, using a ruler
b. Monocular PD, using a pupilometer
c. Binocular PD, using a pupilometer
d. Binocular PD, using a ruler

113. Which best describes a good skull-temple adjustment on a patient?

a. The temples should be as tight as possible, gripping the sides of the head firmly.
b. The temples should be loose on the sides and then begin to bend downward just before reaching the ears.
c. The temples should be snug on the sides and then pass gently over the ears with no additional bend.
d. The temples should lightly meet the head just before the ears and then gently bend around the curve of the ears to rest lightly against the head behind them.

114. What bench tool is commonly used to mount lenses in a modern three-piece frame?

a. End-cutting pliers
b. Compression pliers
c. Numont pliers
d. Half-round pliers

115. When dispensing a new pair of glasses to a patient, it is most important to do which of the following?

a. Verify the new vision at all applicable distances.
b. Invite the patient back to purchase a second or third pair.
c. Give the patient a case and cleaning cloth for the glasses.
d. Invite the patient back for unlimited adjustments.

116. If a patient's vision with the new glasses seems acceptable by the book, but he feels a little disoriented, what should the optician do?

a. Return the patient to the doctor for a prescription recheck.
b. Make a few minor adjustments and then assure the patient he will be fine.
c. Ask the patient to wear his old glasses for the remainder of the day and put on the new ones in the morning after his eyes have rested.
d. Sympathize with the patient, and allow him to vent as long as necessary.

117. Patient education is very important, especially at the point of dispense. What is the most critical thing to impress on a patient who has purchased anti-reflective coating?

a. Treat the lenses with "kid gloves" as they are very delicate.
b. Do not wipe them clean except with the special cloth you will provide.
c. Avoid using alcohol to clean them as it will degrade the coating.
d. Do not leave them in a hot car or in any situation where intense heat can ruin the coating.

118. When a myopic patient is being fitted with stronger lenses, it is natural at first for the glasses to cause what unsettling visual phenomenon?

a. Objects will appear larger than normal.
b. The ground will appear to curve upward.
c. Objects will appear to be shifted to the side.
d. Street curbs will appear to be larger.

119. When fitting young children, what is a good rule of thumb to follow?

a. Make the fitting process into a game to keep their attention.
b. Have lots of toys around the office.
c. Insist on proper, "adult" behavior while you are working with them.
d. Have the parents hold the child still while you take measurements.

120. All glass lenses manufactured in the United States must have what additional procedure(s) completed and documented?

a. A warning label affixed to the eyewear
b. Safety counseling with the patient
c. Heat- or chem-tempering and drop-ball testing
d. Etching the manufacturing lab's monogram in the upper-temporal corner

121. What is the governing body that sets standards for sport-protective eyewear known as?

a. ASTM
b. ANSI
c. OSHA
d. SAE

122. What is the established tolerance for sphere power error in a −6.00 lens?

a. ± 0.15D
b. ± 2%
c. ± 0.33D
d. ± 0.13D

123. A patient comes to you with his or her own frame, asking if you can mount safety lenses into it for use at work. You inspect the frame, and find it to be mechanically sound. What answer do you give the patient?

a. Yes, you can use the frame to mount safety lenses.
b. No, you cannot use the frame to mount safety lenses because it did not come from your shop.
c. No, you cannot use the frame to mount safety lenses because the frame is not marked with "Z87.1."
d. Yes, you can use the frame to mount safety lenses as long as the patient doesn't mind the lens monogram.

124. The use of industrial safety eyewear is ultimately overseen by what governing body?

a. ANSI
b. DOJ
c. GAO
d. OSHA

125. What amount of horizontal prism error is acceptable in a pair of completed eyewear, given the following prescription: OD −3.50 −0.75 X 15, OS −4.00 Sph?

a. 0.67D
b. 2.5 mm
c. 0.33D
d. 1.0 mm

Answer Key and Explanations

1. C: The diopter is the basic unit of measurement for refractive power and is defined as the ability to bend a coherent beam of light by 1 centimeter at a distance of 1 meter from the lens.

2. B: The shape of a plus-power lens is such that the light rays passing through will converge to a point.

3. D: As light passes from one medium (such as air) into a denser one (such as water), it is bent, or refracted.

4. D: Although the UV range begins at around 400 nanometers, it is the shorter wavelengths (below 320 nm) that cause the most damage to the skin. Fortunately, wavelengths shorter than about 290 nm are mostly absorbed by the Earth's atmosphere.

5. A: The focal length of the lens is the distance from its center to the point where the light rays converge to a point, or focus.

6. D: The vertex distance is a measure of how far a corrective lens is placed from the eye and can influence the effective power of the patient's correction if it varies from the distance the doctor used during the eye exam.

7. C: The sphere power of a prescription indicates whether a patient is myopic or hyperopic. Minus values denote myopia, whereas plus values indicate hyperopia.

8. A: Most modern prescriptions are written in minus-cylinder format. Ophthalmologists, simply by tradition, continue to write prescriptions in plus-cylinder format.

9. B: This patient's vision is nearly 20/20 at infinity, but he or she needs correction to read clearly at 35 cm. This condition is known as presbyopia.

10. C: Astigmatism is an out-of-roundness in a patient's cornea and will be oriented in a particular direction. The correction for this in his or her prescription will be a cylindrical value, oriented along a specific axis.

11. A: A sphero-cylinder prescription includes spherical correction for myopia or hyperopia in combination with cylinder power and axis to correct for astigmatism.

12. D: To transpose plus-cylinder prescriptions into minus-cylinder, one must first combine the sphere and cylinder values algebraically, then reverse the sign of the cylinder value, and finally invert the axis by 90 degrees.

13. B: To transpose a plus-cylinder prescription with an add into near-vision only for ordering, one must first combine the sphere and cylinder values algebraically, reverse the sign of the cylinder value, then invert the axis by 90 degrees, and finally combine the add power with the sphere power.

14. C: Rarely seen today, the lenticular lens was often used with aphakic patients (without natural crystalline lens or implanted IOLs). It had an odd appearance, but it did accomplish the goal of being lighter in weight than a full-field +16.00 lens would have been.

15. D: Toric lenses have two curvatures on the back side: one to correct for myopia or hyperopia and the other to correct astigmatism.

16. B: The surface power of a lens is calculated directly from its front and back curvatures, assuming a refractive index of 1.50.

17. C: The refractive index of polycarbonate is greater than mid-index (1.56) but less than high index (1.60 and 1.67), generally measured at about 1.58.

18. D: The scale measuring optical clarity was developed by German physicist Ernst Abbe and still bears his name.

19. A: The spherical equivalent of a prescription is found by halving the cylinder power (in this case, first transposing the prescription into minus-cylinder format, combining sphere and cylinder algebraically, changing the sign of the cylinder, and inverting the axis 90 degrees, resulting in +1.25 −3.50 X 81) and combining it with the sphere power: −1.75 +1.25 = −0.50. The axis is disregarded.

20. C: Along the line of the cylinder axis, the cylinder power has no effect. Its full effect is found 90 degrees from that axis. At 45 degrees from the axis, exactly half of the cylinder power comes into play, which in this case is −1.00, precisely canceling out the sphere power of +1.00, leaving the lens plano in that meridian.

21. B: Transposing from minus-cylinder to plus-cylinder is accomplished by first combining the sphere and cylinder powers algebraically, then reversing the sign of the cylinder, and finally inverting the axis by 90 degrees.

22. D: The Prentice formula (prism = [decentration x power] / 10) is applied here as follows: amount of decentration = 3 mm, lens power = 4 diopters—3 x 4 = 12, divided by 10 = 1.2 diopters of prism induced.

23. C: Because unwanted vertical prism is a relative value, its effect is measured on the weaker lens of the two, which determines the end effect on the patient.

24. A: Focal length (in meters) is the reciprocal of dioptric power. In this case, the conversion formula would read 1 divided by 0.4 meters, or 2.50. Because the lens has a measurable focal length, it must be a plus lens.

25. D: The vertex formula is Dc = D / (1-dD), where D is the written power, d is the vertex deviation in meters, and Dc is the resulting change in effective power. Therefore, 12.00 / (1 – [.005 x 12]), or 12 / (1-.06), or 12 / .94 = 12.77 for the effective power at an 18 mm vertex distance because a plus lens always increases with the vertex. The increase of 0.77 should be subtracted, ordering a compensated power of +11.23.

26. B: The progressive-addition multifocal has a power corridor down the center, which smoothly increases the power of the lens toward the bottom.

27. C: Although this archaic lens style is seldom used anymore, it did feature a near visual field that spanned the entire lower portion of the lens.

28. A: Image jump happens when the eye is forced to quickly transition from one lens curvature to another. Even the blended bifocal has an unpleasant "blur zone" at the edge of the add power, which suddenly shifts the image. Progressive lenses eliminate this problem as nearly as possible.

29. D: The higher index of refraction of flint glass is what causes an inlaid segment to produce a higher lens power as light passes into it from the lower-index crown glass around it.

30. B: The presbyope who needs crisp near vision at multiple places in the visual field would benefit most from an occupational multifocal such as the double-D bifocal, giving him more than one functional area for close work.

31. D: Near variable focus lenses are a type of progressive lens in which the entire upper portion of the lens is configured for intermediate use. (The add corridor delivers the remaining power for near vision at the bottom.)

32. A: Although Trivex does have several advantages in the way of impact-resistance and optical clarity, its refractive index is only 1.53 and so will always produce a thicker lens than materials such as polycarbonate and polyurethanes.

33. D: Most newer lens materials require coatings to reduce scratch resistance, and those coatings are often vulnerable to chemical corrosion. Crown glass by its nature is impervious to most chemicals.

34. C: Either polycarbonate or Trivex would satisfy the impact resistance necessary for a patient under the age of 18, but polycarbonate is the much more affordable option of the two. It will also produce a much thinner lens than Trivex.

35. B: The index of refraction of a material is a measure of its ability to slow down light passing through it. It represents the speed of light in air divided by the speed of light through the material. Refraction occurs at the boundary between the two.

36. D: Although the thinnest lens would be produced by using a 1.71 index material, the resulting optical quality will suffer enough to make the visual clarity unacceptable to the patient. The better-balanced choice would be to use a 1.67 index material, which is nearly as thin but has better optics.

37. C: Diplopia is a condition in which the eyes cannot fuse the binocular information into a single image. Prism can be used to shift the light in the right direction to assist the eyes in merging the two images.

38. B: Whereas a prism will shift the resulting image in the direction of the prism's apex, the light itself is actually bent toward the base of the prism.

39. D: Decentering a minus lens further from the nose increases the nasal edge thickness and induces base-in prism. In this case, the Prentice formula is inverted algebraically to solve for decentration: decentration = (prism x 10) divided by power. This applies as (2 prism diopters x 10) divided by −3.75 diopters of lens power = 5.33.

40. B: This type of prism is known as "slab-off" prism and is applied to only the lower portion of the most-minus lens. Properly applied, it will result in eliminating the vertical imbalance when the patient lowers his or her eyes to read through the lower areas of the lens.

41. A: Vertical prism error is always measured at the weaker of the two lenses, which in this case is the left, because at the 90th meridian nearly all of the OD cylinder power comes into play, creating a vertical power of −5.00 in that lens. So, 1/3 diopter of deviation is the acceptable limit.

42. C: This patient may be able to see well-enough without prism correction but applying it will palliatively reduce eye strain and eye fatigue.

43. D: Whereas the aqueous humor fills the smaller anterior chamber of the eye, the much-larger posterior chamber is occupied by the vitreous humor, which is responsible for helping the eye hold its shape.

44. C: With a power of about +43.00 diopters, the cornea is responsible for the majority of the refraction performed by the eye, similar to the large "objective" lens at the front of a refracting telescope.

45. B: Rods are responsible for reproducing black-and-white images, but the cones give us our perception of colors.

46. B: The puncta are the tiny holes near the nasal corners of the eye and act as little vacuums to draw away the excess tears.

47. D: A patient with anisometropia will have a prescription that varies wildly from one eye to the other, such as OD −1.50, OS −11.00.

48. A: The hyperopic eye is able to see well at long distances but is unable to focus on objects which are nearby.

49. C: Myopia results from the refractive elements of the eye being too strong or the eye being too elongated. As a result, the light is focused at a point shorter than the distance to the retina.

50. D: Mixed astigmatism is the result of an aspheric lens or cornea bringing light into focus at more than one point, neither of which falls precisely on the retina.

51. B: The normal onset of presbyopia occurs shortly after the age of 40 as the crystalline lens loses enough of its ability to change shape that the patient is no longer able to focus on nearby objects. This will often manifest most obviously at the end of a day spent straining to do so.

52. C: While it does not have the hypoallergenic properties of stainless steel, monel (an alloy of nickel, copper, and manganese) is rigid, less expensive than gold, and easier to work with than aluminum, making it the most popular metal frame material.

53. D: The semi-rimless frame has a solid frame partway around the lenses and holds them tightly by means of a stretched nylon filament around the remainder of the circumference.

54. A: Optyl may be heated and/or stretched, and made wet or dry, but when cooling down it rapidly, it crystallizes and passes through a very brittle phase, during which the material should not be moved.

55. D: Zyl (cellulose acetate) frames hold their shape and color extremely well, are hypoallergenic, and can be heated without undue shrinkage.

56. B: Although polycarbonate has very high impact resistance and is acceptable in most situations, Trivex is slightly tougher.

57. A: Although progressive lenses offer a number of advantages, their inescapable peripheral distortion is not one of them. All of them suffer from this to some degree, which reduces the effective visual field in even the best designs.

58. C: This lens offers variable areas of focus over the intermediate to near ranges, deliberately ignoring the distance vision.

59. B: The middle portion of a trifocal add is generally half as strong as the lower portion.

60. C: Polarized lenses utilize a bonded laminate on the surface, which permits only direct light rays and cancels light from reflected surfaces.

61. D: Although protection from UV exposure is important, it is often already inherent in many modern lens materials. Anti-reflective coatings simply increase the optical clarity of any lens, helping the patient see more clearly.

62. A: Although photochromatic lenses can be beneficial in a variety of situations, many patients do not care for them, they are limited in availability, and they will never provide sun protection equal to that of a polarized lens.

63. B: The primary drawback to CR-39 lenses is that they will shatter and are therefore unsafe to use in sports applications or children's eyewear.

64. D: The cylinder power is manifested most strongly 90 degrees away from the axis, which makes for the maximum thickness at OD 137 degrees and OS 39 degrees.

65. C: Use of a semi-rimless frame will require the entire lens to be thickened up to produce a minimum thickness along the bottom edge, where a groove will have to hold a nylon filament.

66. D: As its name implies, a well-fit saddle bridge mates with the nose like a saddle on a horse, spreading the weight consistently all around the bridge of the nose.

67. B: The correct method in choosing base curve is to first find the sphere equivalent of the prescription, which is sphere power + ½ cylinder power, or +1.00 in this case. This number is added to the nominal +6.00 (the average curvature of the human eye) to give +7.00, the closest manufactured base curve typically being +7.25. Using this base curve will produce an average back surface curvature closest to −6.00, roughly paralleling the surface of the eye to produce the most natural vision.

68. C: Polarized lenses are good for many things, but they often cancel out digital LCD displays, which work by electrically polarizing the liquid crystals.

69. A: Most photochromatic lenses rely on direct exposure to UV light to change, and the glass of the car windows screens out most of this UV light. Thus, the tint of a photochromatic lens will be very light behind the wheel.

70. D: Anti-reflective coating is designed to eliminate the confusing extra images produced by multiple reflected light sources all trying to pass through the lens and creating their own reflections at the same time.

71. C: The anti-fatigue lens styles have a small "bump" of power at the bottom for early pre-presbyopes. This can often stave off the problems associated with emerging presbyopia, by slightly easing the eye strain first experienced in the near visual field after a long day.

72. B: Double-D lenses are available with equal or unequal add powers, which can be critical if, for example, he needs near vision down below, but the eaves are 24 inches away.

73. D: With all the choices in progressive lenses, we no longer need to tell the patient to choose a larger frame. Because she has already chosen the frame she wants, the next step is to narrow down the progressive choices to the ones that have corridors that fit comfortably within the frame, allowing her full near power.

74. C: This patient's primary issue is the thickness and weight of the lenses. An aspheric design can be the best way to dramatically reduce both.

75. B: The manufacturer's reference point, on the 180-line directly underneath the fitting cross, is the point at which prism, either prescribed or accidental, should be measured.

76. D: The amount of any imbalance is measured at the weaker of the two lenses. Therefore, it is critical to begin by centering the lensometer on the stronger lens.

77. A: Visible misalignment of the bifocal segments, often (regrettably) dismissed by the optician as trivial, will be immediately noticeable and perpetually annoying to the patient, not to mention being a poor advertisement for the practice.

78. B: Often referred to as "four-point alignment," this is the practice of squaring up a frame so that it has no excessive tilt or wrap, the lenses are in coplanar alignment with each other, the temples are parallel, and the frame contacts the table at all four corners.

79. D: A photometer bathes the lenses in UV light, which will promptly cause a photochromatic lens to darken or reveal the absence of this property.

80. D: If the lab accidentally installed the lenses in the wrong frame, nothing else will matter. It is easy to concentrate on the optics or the lens cosmetics, but if you hand the completed work to the patient, and he or she states, "That's not what I ordered," the entire process falls apart.

81. C: The power drum of the lensometer is rotated until the image in the eyepiece comes into focus, and the power of the lens is then read from the circular scale wrapped around the drum.

82. A: A cylindrical lens will be brought to focus at two different points, one of which is the sphere power, and the difference between the two is the cylinder power.

83. D: While lower powers may be acceptably read from the front, the most accurate power reading on a segmented multifocal will always be taken from the back side.

84. B: The spherometer, often called the lens clock (or sometimes the Geneva Lens Measure), is a small tool with a dial gauge that is used to measure the curvature of a lens. Holding the three pins perpendicular to the lens, the pins are pressed against the center of the lens surface, and the curvature is read on the dial.

85. C: Rotating the power drum all the way plus-ward allows the operator to bring the drum back until the image comes into focus at the most-plus power, at which point the axis wheel is rotated to bring the thin mires into alignment. The sphere power is then read at the power drum.

86. C: Although newer lensometers have a prism compensator built onto the rear of the eyepiece assembly, older models may need to have auxiliary prism rings available. These are little disks with prism values (typically 3D, 6D, and 9D), which are inserted into a receptacle directly behind the eyepiece, displace the image by exactly that amount.

87. A: To determine the exact amount of prism that was ground into a bifocal lens, the targeted placement for the optical center must first be established—in this case, its relationship to the location of the segment.

88. D: The manufacturer-specified distance circle is the approved spot to verify the distance power of a progressive lens.

89. B: The frame table's purpose is to maintain a level relationship between right and left lenses to insure the absence of vertical imbalance. With the table left in place, the right lens should normally center in the eyepiece just like the left lens.

90. C: The eyepiece adjustment is there to account for small differences in vision between opticians. Leaving it unadjusted could result in all the powers seeming to be off by as much as 0.25D. Never begin work without first focusing the eyepiece.

91. D: Although a typical patient's eyes do converge about 3 mm when focused at the near point, the more accurate method is to set the pupilometer to near range (35 cm) and then take a reading.

92. A: The lens caliper is a simple device that gently pinches the lens between nylon-tipped jaws and reads the thickness on a vernier scale. More complicated versions come equipped with a dial gauge for more accurate measurements.

93. C: A lens that is being squeezed too tightly within a frame will display stress patterns in a polariscope. These are danger zones where the lens may shatter if the stress is not relieved. A properly heat-tempered glass lens will also show a uniform pattern of distributed stresses throughout the lens.

94. B: The C-gauge, or circumference-gauge, is a device that can measure the exact circumference of the lens using a small tape rule stretched around it. Armed with this piece of information, the lab will easily be able to reproduce a lens of the exact size needed for the patient's frame.

95. B: The distometer is a small instrument used to measure between the surface of a patient's (closed) eye and the back of the lenses, known as the vertex distance.

96. D: A-R coated lenses are susceptible to heat and can easily be crazed by the high temperatures of a frame warmer. To be sure they will not be destroyed, they should be removed prior to applying any heat.

97. C: The small pointer that reads the power on the drum often has a small amount of adjustment available to it. Simply focusing the lensometer at plano, loosening the pointer, and retightening it to read at zero may solve this problem.

98. A: The entire instrument should not need daily cleaning. Simply keeping the instrument shielded from dust accumulation will provide the greatest benefit, that of reducing the need to clean dust from the optics.

99. D: This is an example of a vertex error, similar to what happens when a high-power lens is moved closer or further from the eye. Adjusting the lens stop in or out will change the vertex—in this case, the distance from the lens to the primary optics of the lensometer—and correct the progressive error at high powers.

100. B: Although disposable paper shields are available for certain instruments, they are impractical in most situations. Using an alcohol wipe after each patient is the simplest way to insure against the spreading of disease.

101. C: Although contact lenses can be useful in sports activities, this patient has obviously elected to stick with glasses. A padded sport frame with photochromatic lenses would stay on better, protect the patient best from occasionally getting hit by the ball, and do double duty for daytime and nighttime play.

102. A: The piano keyboard falls around the 24"–32" range from the pianist's eyes, squarely within intermediate territory. Because this patient does not rely on reading music, there is no need for near vision to be addressed, and he or she may benefit most from a pair of intermediate-vision-only glasses.

103. D: Although not cosmetically flashy, the CRT lens, with its 14 mm-tall intermediate area, would give this patient a nice picture-window view of a clear computer screen while leaving him plenty of crisp distance vision for reading labels in the warehouse.

104. C: This patient needs to have good near vision in more than one place. Standard multifocals all put that portion of the lens at the bottom, whereas occupational lenses allow the patient to also have it at the top.

105. D: Near-variable focus lenses will give the patient an upper half dedicated to her computer screen while still allowing her to see the keyboard or some printed material with ease.

106. A: A trifocal is intended to be fit at the bottom of the patient's pupil. This must be tempered by the patient's wearing history and stated preferences as well as any specialized situation that demands customization of the fit.

107. B: The bottom of a frame should tilt inward toward the face, typically at an angle of 5 to 10 degrees. This is considered normal pantoscopic tilt and will put the reading area of the lenses in a much more accessible place.

108. C: The Numont pliers, with their transverse channel near the tip, will solidly hold the end piece of a metal frame still while the angling pliers induce a downward angle at either the remaining frame corner or the hinge.

109. B: Placement of the optical center (OC) is generally standardized with pairs of lined multifocals and progressive lenses. Although it can sometimes be helpful to raise the OCs on polycarbonate and high-index lenses (to place the clearest vision directly in front of the pupil), it is absolutely essential to match the opposite lens's OC position on a single-lens replacement of a lined multifocal.

110. D: You should always begin progressive verification by noting the optical center placement at the MRP prior to completing any remaining steps that will be rendered moot if the lenses show unacceptable vertical imbalance.

111. C: Although both lenses technically have an unacceptable amount of induced prism, the left lens falls within 1 mm of the specified PD and is therefore acceptable. The right lens must be remade (Prentice formula: [3 mm x −4.00] /10 = 1.2D prism), but it is up to the optician's discretion as to whether to reorder both lenses (due to a total binocular induced prism of 1.675) in hopes of a better result.

112. B: The power corridors of progressive lenses are narrow enough that a slight deviation in horizontal placement can be enough to sink an otherwise successful fit. Therefore, the most accurate monocular PD should be used, and that is obtained with a corneal reflective pupilometer.

113. D: Proper temple fit can make or break a new pair of glasses, and this method will insure lasting comfort for the patient.

114. B: Most modern three-piece or "rimless" frames are assembled with compression mountings, which require specialized compression pliers to squeeze pins into bushings for a tight assembly.

115. A: Although extras like cases and cloths make a patient feel good, and he or she should always be encouraged to return whenever needed, delivery of a new pair of glasses is never complete until the optician has verified that the glasses function as they should.

116. C: If a patient has been struggling with inadequate correction, his eyes have been trying to accommodate and failing. After the patient has slept for the night, his eyes will be relaxed and ready for the proper correction.

117. D: Although gentle cleaning is good to encourage, most patients will do this with little prompting. What they will probably not know is how easily destroyed the coating is by excessive heat and how quickly this can happen in a 150-degree car parked in the sun.

118. B: The effect of a stronger minus prescription will always be that objects appear to be shifted inward toward the center of the lens. This is most noticeable at the ground or floor, where the patient will feel as if he or she is walking uphill. The effect will fade over a few days.

119. A: Most children have short attention spans, but if you can make the process something fun for them, with "magic tricks," like making one pupilometer image "vanish" while the other suddenly appears, you will not only accomplish what you need to, but you will have a happy patient for life.

120. C: Glass lenses must be hardened by heat-tempering or chem-tempering and must survive a 5/8" steel ball dropped from a height of 50 inches. These results must be documented and kept for 3 years.

121. A: Standards for sports-related products are designed by the American Society for Testing Materials (ASTM). Section F803 is the area pertaining to protective eyewear used in sports, and all approved sports frames will bear the mark "ASTM F803."

122. D: ANSI Z80.1-2015 specifies that 13/100ths of a diopter in power is the acceptable limit for error, up to powers of ± 6.50D. Above that, the tolerance changes to 2%.

123. C: No frame materials that have not passed Z87.1 testing may be used in manufacturing safety eyewear. Lens monogramming is required but does not excuse the use of a non-Z87.1 frame.

124. D: Industrial safety eyewear, and its use in the workplace, is loosely policed by the Occupational Safety and Health Administration (OSHA).

125. B: Above powers of ± 2.75, a total of 2.5 mm deviation from the specified binocular PD is technically acceptable, regardless of how much horizontal prism is induced.

How to Overcome Test Anxiety

Just the thought of taking a test is enough to make most people a little nervous. A test is an important event that can have a long-term impact on your future, so it's important to take it seriously and it's natural to feel anxious about performing well. But just because anxiety is normal, that doesn't mean that it's helpful in test taking, or that you should simply accept it as part of your life. Anxiety can have a variety of effects. These effects can be mild, like making you feel slightly nervous, or severe, like blocking your ability to focus or remember even a simple detail.

If you experience test anxiety—whether severe or mild—it's important to know how to beat it. To discover this, first you need to understand what causes test anxiety.

Causes of Test Anxiety

While we often think of anxiety as an uncontrollable emotional state, it can actually be caused by simple, practical things. One of the most common causes of test anxiety is that a person does not feel adequately prepared for their test. This feeling can be the result of many different issues such as poor study habits or lack of organization, but the most common culprit is time management. Starting to study too late, failing to organize your study time to cover all of the material, or being distracted while you study will mean that you're not well prepared for the test. This may lead to cramming the night before, which will cause you to be physically and mentally exhausted for the test. Poor time management also contributes to feelings of stress, fear, and hopelessness as you realize you are not well prepared but don't know what to do about it.

Other times, test anxiety is not related to your preparation for the test but comes from unresolved fear. This may be a past failure on a test, or poor performance on tests in general. It may come from comparing yourself to others who seem to be performing better or from the stress of living up to expectations. Anxiety may be driven by fears of the future—how failure on this test would affect your educational and career goals. These fears are often completely irrational, but they can still negatively impact your test performance.

Review Video: 3 Reasons You Have Test Anxiety
Visit mometrix.com/academy and enter code: 428468

Elements of Test Anxiety

As mentioned earlier, test anxiety is considered to be an emotional state, but it has physical and mental components as well. Sometimes you may not even realize that you are suffering from test anxiety until you notice the physical symptoms. These can include trembling hands, rapid heartbeat, sweating, nausea, and tense muscles. Extreme anxiety may lead to fainting or vomiting. Obviously, any of these symptoms can have a negative impact on testing. It is important to recognize them as soon as they begin to occur so that you can address the problem before it damages your performance.

Review Video: 3 Ways to Tell You Have Test Anxiety
Visit mometrix.com/academy and enter code: 927847

The mental components of test anxiety include trouble focusing and inability to remember learned information. During a test, your mind is on high alert, which can help you recall information and stay focused for an extended period of time. However, anxiety interferes with your mind's natural processes, causing you to blank out, even on the questions you know well. The strain of testing during anxiety makes it difficult to stay focused, especially on a test that may take several hours. Extreme anxiety can take a huge mental toll, making it difficult not only to recall test information but even to understand the test questions or pull your thoughts together.

Review Video: How Test Anxiety Affects Memory
Visit mometrix.com/academy and enter code: 609003

Effects of Test Anxiety

Test anxiety is like a disease—if left untreated, it will get progressively worse. Anxiety leads to poor performance, and this reinforces the feelings of fear and failure, which in turn lead to poor performances on subsequent tests. It can grow from a mild nervousness to a crippling condition. If allowed to progress, test anxiety can have a big impact on your schooling, and consequently on your future.

Test anxiety can spread to other parts of your life. Anxiety on tests can become anxiety in any stressful situation, and blanking on a test can turn into panicking in a job situation. But fortunately, you don't have to let anxiety rule your testing and determine your grades. There are a number of relatively simple steps you can take to move past anxiety and function normally on a test and in the rest of life.

Review Video: How Test Anxiety Impacts Your Grades
Visit mometrix.com/academy and enter code: 939819

Physical Steps for Beating Test Anxiety

While test anxiety is a serious problem, the good news is that it can be overcome. It doesn't have to control your ability to think and remember information. While it may take time, you can begin taking steps today to beat anxiety.

Just as your first hint that you may be struggling with anxiety comes from the physical symptoms, the first step to treating it is also physical. Rest is crucial for having a clear, strong mind. If you are tired, it is much easier to give in to anxiety. But if you establish good sleep habits, your body and mind will be ready to perform optimally, without the strain of exhaustion. Additionally, sleeping well helps you to retain information better, so you're more likely to recall the answers when you see the test questions.

Getting good sleep means more than going to bed on time. It's important to allow your brain time to relax. Take study breaks from time to time so it doesn't get overworked, and don't study right before bed. Take time to rest your mind before trying to rest your body, or you may find it difficult to fall asleep.

Review Video: The Importance of Sleep for Your Brain
Visit mometrix.com/academy and enter code: 319338

Along with sleep, other aspects of physical health are important in preparing for a test. Good nutrition is vital for good brain function. Sugary foods and drinks may give a burst of energy but this burst is followed by a crash, both physically and emotionally. Instead, fuel your body with protein and vitamin-rich foods.

Also, drink plenty of water. Dehydration can lead to headaches and exhaustion, especially if your brain is already under stress from the rigors of the test. Particularly if your test is a long one, drink water during the breaks. And if possible, take an energy-boosting snack to eat between sections.

Review Video: How Diet Can Affect your Mood
Visit mometrix.com/academy and enter code: 624317

Along with sleep and diet, a third important part of physical health is exercise. Maintaining a steady workout schedule is helpful, but even taking 5-minute study breaks to walk can help get your blood pumping faster and clear your head. Exercise also releases endorphins, which contribute to a positive feeling and can help combat test anxiety.

When you nurture your physical health, you are also contributing to your mental health. If your body is healthy, your mind is much more likely to be healthy as well. So take time to rest, nourish your body with healthy food and water, and get moving as much as possible. Taking these physical steps will make you stronger and more able to take the mental steps necessary to overcome test anxiety.

Mental Steps for Beating Test Anxiety

Working on the mental side of test anxiety can be more challenging, but as with the physical side, there are clear steps you can take to overcome it. As mentioned earlier, test anxiety often stems from lack of preparation, so the obvious solution is to prepare for the test. Effective studying may be the most important weapon you have for beating test anxiety, but you can and should employ several other mental tools to combat fear.

First, boost your confidence by reminding yourself of past success—tests or projects that you aced. If you're putting as much effort into preparing for this test as you did for those, there's no reason you should expect to fail here. Work hard to prepare; then trust your preparation.

Second, surround yourself with encouraging people. It can be helpful to find a study group, but be sure that the people you're around will encourage a positive attitude. If you spend time with others who are anxious or cynical, this will only contribute to your own anxiety. Look for others who are motivated to study hard from a desire to succeed, not from a fear of failure.

Third, reward yourself. A test is physically and mentally tiring, even without anxiety, and it can be helpful to have something to look forward to. Plan an activity following the test, regardless of the outcome, such as going to a movie or getting ice cream.

When you are taking the test, if you find yourself beginning to feel anxious, remind yourself that you know the material. Visualize successfully completing the test. Then take a few deep, relaxing breaths and return to it. Work through the questions carefully but with confidence, knowing that you are capable of succeeding.

Developing a healthy mental approach to test taking will also aid in other areas of life. Test anxiety affects more than just the actual test—it can be damaging to your mental health and even contribute to depression. It's important to beat test anxiety before it becomes a problem for more than testing.

Review Video: Test Anxiety and Depression
Visit mometrix.com/academy and enter code: 904704

Study Strategy

Being prepared for the test is necessary to combat anxiety, but what does being prepared look like? You may study for hours on end and still not feel prepared. What you need is a strategy for test prep. The next few pages outline our recommended steps to help you plan out and conquer the challenge of preparation.

Step 1: Scope Out the Test

Learn everything you can about the format (multiple choice, essay, etc.) and what will be on the test. Gather any study materials, course outlines, or sample exams that may be available. Not only will this help you to prepare, but knowing what to expect can help to alleviate test anxiety.

Step 2: Map Out the Material

Look through the textbook or study guide and make note of how many chapters or sections it has. Then divide these over the time you have. For example, if a book has 15 chapters and you have five days to study, you need to cover three chapters each day. Even better, if you have the time, leave an extra day at the end for overall review after you have gone through the material in depth.

If time is limited, you may need to prioritize the material. Look through it and make note of which sections you think you already have a good grasp on, and which need review. While you are studying, skim quickly through the familiar sections and take more time on the challenging parts. Write out your plan so you don't get lost as you go. Having a written plan also helps you feel more in control of the study, so anxiety is less likely to arise from feeling overwhelmed at the amount to cover.

Step 3: Gather Your Tools

Decide what study method works best for you. Do you prefer to highlight in the book as you study and then go back over the highlighted portions? Or do you type out notes of the important information? Or is it helpful to make flashcards that you can carry with you? Assemble the pens, index cards, highlighters, post-it notes, and any other materials you may need so you won't be distracted by getting up to find things while you study.

If you're having a hard time retaining the information or organizing your notes, experiment with different methods. For example, try color-coding by subject with colored pens, highlighters, or post-it notes. If you learn better by hearing, try recording yourself reading your notes so you can listen while in the car, working out, or simply sitting at your desk. Ask a friend to quiz you from your flashcards, or try teaching someone the material to solidify it in your mind.

Step 4: Create Your Environment

It's important to avoid distractions while you study. This includes both the obvious distractions like visitors and the subtle distractions like an uncomfortable chair (or a too-comfortable couch that makes you want to fall asleep). Set up the best study environment possible: good lighting and a comfortable work area. If background music helps you focus, you may want to turn it on, but otherwise keep the room quiet. If you are using a computer to take notes, be sure you don't have any other windows open, especially applications like social media, games, or anything else that could distract you. Silence your phone and turn off notifications. Be sure to keep water close by so you stay hydrated while you study (but avoid unhealthy drinks and snacks).

Also, take into account the best time of day to study. Are you freshest first thing in the morning? Try to set aside some time then to work through the material. Is your mind clearer in the afternoon or evening? Schedule your study session then. Another method is to study at the same time of day that you will take the test, so that your brain gets used to working on the material at that time and will be ready to focus at test time.

Step 5: Study!

Once you have done all the study preparation, it's time to settle into the actual studying. Sit down, take a few moments to settle your mind so you can focus, and begin to follow your study plan. Don't give in to distractions or let yourself procrastinate. This is your time to prepare so you'll be ready to fearlessly approach the test. Make the most of the time and stay focused.

Of course, you don't want to burn out. If you study too long you may find that you're not retaining the information very well. Take regular study breaks. For example, taking five minutes out of every hour to walk briskly, breathing deeply and swinging your arms, can help your mind stay fresh.

As you get to the end of each chapter or section, it's a good idea to do a quick review. Remind yourself of what you learned and work on any difficult parts. When you feel that you've mastered the material, move on to the next part. At the end of your study session, briefly skim through your notes again.

But while review is helpful, cramming last minute is NOT. If at all possible, work ahead so that you won't need to fit all your study into the last day. Cramming overloads your brain with more information than it can process and retain, and your tired mind may struggle to recall even previously learned information when it is overwhelmed with last-minute study. Also, the urgent nature of cramming and the stress placed on your brain contribute to anxiety. You'll be more likely to go to the test feeling unprepared and having trouble thinking clearly.

So don't cram, and don't stay up late before the test, even just to review your notes at a leisurely pace. Your brain needs rest more than it needs to go over the information again. In fact, plan to finish your studies by noon or early afternoon the day before the test. Give your brain the rest of the day to relax or focus on other things, and get a good night's sleep. Then you will be fresh for the test and better able to recall what you've studied.

Step 6: Take a Practice Test

Many courses offer sample tests, either online or in the study materials. This is an excellent resource to check whether you have mastered the material, as well as to prepare for the test format and environment.

Check the test format ahead of time: the number of questions, the type (multiple choice, free response, etc.), and the time limit. Then create a plan for working through them. For example, if you have 30 minutes to take a 60-question test, your limit is 30 seconds per question. Spend less time on the questions you know well so that you can take more time on the difficult ones.

If you have time to take several practice tests, take the first one open book, with no time limit. Work through the questions at your own pace and make sure you fully understand them. Gradually work up to taking a test under test conditions: sit at a desk with all study materials put away and set a timer. Pace yourself to make sure you finish the test with time to spare and go back to check your answers if you have time.

After each test, check your answers. On the questions you missed, be sure you understand why you missed them. Did you misread the question (tests can use tricky wording)? Did you forget the information? Or was it something you hadn't learned? Go back and study any shaky areas that the practice tests reveal.

Taking these tests not only helps with your grade, but also aids in combating test anxiety. If you're already used to the test conditions, you're less likely to worry about it, and working through tests until you're scoring well gives you a confidence boost. Go through the practice tests until you feel comfortable, and then you can go into the test knowing that you're ready for it.

Test Tips

On test day, you should be confident, knowing that you've prepared well and are ready to answer the questions. But aside from preparation, there are several test day strategies you can employ to maximize your performance.

First, as stated before, get a good night's sleep the night before the test (and for several nights before that, if possible). Go into the test with a fresh, alert mind rather than staying up late to study.

Try not to change too much about your normal routine on the day of the test. It's important to eat a nutritious breakfast, but if you normally don't eat breakfast at all, consider eating just a protein bar. If you're a coffee drinker, go ahead and have your normal coffee. Just make sure you time it so that the caffeine doesn't wear off right in the middle of your test. Avoid sugary beverages, and drink enough water to stay hydrated but not so much that you need a restroom break 10 minutes into the test. If your test isn't first thing in the morning, consider going for a walk or doing a light workout before the test to get your blood flowing.

Allow yourself enough time to get ready, and leave for the test with plenty of time to spare so you won't have the anxiety of scrambling to arrive in time. Another reason to be early is to select a good seat. It's helpful to sit away from doors and windows, which can be distracting. Find a good seat, get out your supplies, and settle your mind before the test begins.

When the test begins, start by going over the instructions carefully, even if you already know what to expect. Make sure you avoid any careless mistakes by following the directions.

Then begin working through the questions, pacing yourself as you've practiced. If you're not sure on an answer, don't spend too much time on it, and don't let it shake your confidence. Either skip it and come back later, or eliminate as many wrong answers as possible and guess among the remaining ones. Don't dwell on these questions as you continue—put them out of your mind and focus on what lies ahead.

Be sure to read all of the answer choices, even if you're sure the first one is the right answer. Sometimes you'll find a better one if you keep reading. But don't second-guess yourself if you do immediately know the answer. Your gut instinct is usually right. Don't let test anxiety rob you of the information you know.

If you have time at the end of the test (and if the test format allows), go back and review your answers. Be cautious about changing any, since your first instinct tends to be correct, but make sure you didn't misread any of the questions or accidentally mark the wrong answer choice. Look over any you skipped and make an educated guess.

At the end, leave the test feeling confident. You've done your best, so don't waste time worrying about your performance or wishing you could change anything. Instead, celebrate the successful completion of this test. And finally, use this test to learn how to deal with anxiety even better next time.

Review Video: 5 Tips to Beat Test Anxiety
Visit mometrix.com/academy and enter code: 570656

Important Qualification

Not all anxiety is created equal. If your test anxiety is causing major issues in your life beyond the classroom or testing center, or if you are experiencing troubling physical symptoms related to your anxiety, it may be a sign of a serious physiological or psychological condition. If this sounds like your situation, we strongly encourage you to seek professional help.

Thank You

We at Mometrix would like to extend our heartfelt thanks to you, our friend and patron, for allowing us to play a part in your journey. It is a privilege to serve people from all walks of life who are unified in their commitment to building the best future they can for themselves.

The preparation you devote to these important testing milestones may be the most valuable educational opportunity you have for making a real difference in your life. We encourage you to put your heart into it—that feeling of succeeding, overcoming, and yes, conquering will be well worth the hours you've invested.

We want to hear your story, your struggles and your successes, and if you see any opportunities for us to improve our materials so we can help others even more effectively in the future, please share that with us as well. **The team at Mometrix would be absolutely thrilled to hear from you!** So please, send us an email (support@mometrix.com) and let's stay in touch.

If you'd like some additional help, check out these other resources we offer for your exam: http://mometrixflashcards.com/NOCE

Additional Bonus Material

Due to our efforts to try to keep this book to a manageable length, we've created a link that will give you access to all of your additional bonus material:

mometrix.com/bonus948/noce